ALLERGY-FREE KIDS

ALLERGY-FREE KIDS

KIDS

THE SCIENCE-BASED APPROACH TO PREVENTING FOOD ALLERGIES

Robin Nixon Pompa

Foreword by Gideon Lack, MD,
Professor of Paediatric Allergy, King's College London,
and principal researcher behind the allergy
intervention studies LEAP and EAT

wm

WILLIAM MORROW
An Imprint of HarperCollins*Publishers*

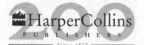

HarperCollins books may be purchased for educational, business, or sales promotional use. For information, please email the Special Markets Department at SPsales@harpercollins.com.

FIRST EDITION

Allergen icons by OSSOBUKO/Shutterstock, Inc.

Library of Congress Cataloging-in-Publication Data

Names: Pompa, Robin Nixon, author.
Title: Allergy-free kids : the science-based approach to preventing food
    allergies / Robin Nixon Pompa ; foreword by Gideon Lack, MD, Professor
    of Paediatric Allergy, King's College London and principal researcher
    behind the allergy intervention studies LEAP and EAT.
Description: First edition. | New York, NY : William Morrow, [2017]
Identifiers: LCCN 2016038525 | ISBN 9780062440686 (hardback)
Subjects: LCSH: Allergy in children--Prevention--Popular works. | Allergy in
    children--Treatment--Popular works. | Food allergy--Prevention--Popular
    works. | BISAC: HEALTH & FITNESS / Allergies. | FAMILY & RELATIONSHIPS /
    Parenting / General. | COOKING / Health & Healing / Allergy.
Classification: LCC RJ386 .P66 2017 | DDC 618.92/9750654--dc23 LC record
    available at https://lccn.loc.gov/2016038525

ISBN 978-0-06-244068-6

17 18 19 20 21 LSC 10 9 8 7 6 5 4 3 2 1

To Clara, Grady, and Arthur

Contents

Foreword

My immediate reaction to this book was that it would help my patients implement some of the clinical messages that have come out of my research.

For more than a decade now, my colleagues and I have been investigating the rise in food allergies, and we came to the conclusion that there was insufficient evidence to support delayed weaning of allergenic (allergy-causing) foods in young babies. We had always been taught that infants' immune systems needed time to mature before being challenged with potentially dangerous food allergens that could eventually lead to allergic reactions. The logic seemed sound, but there was insufficient evidence to back this up. Guidelines issued in the United States in 2000 recommended avoiding the introduction of nuts, eggs, and other major allergens until late toddlerhood, and similar guidelines in the United Kingdom suggested that peanut ought to be avoided in young infants' diets. Nevertheless, over more than a decade and a half of avoidance, the rate of food allergy continued to rise. There were, however, some notable exceptions to this.

For example, my colleagues and I heard from Israeli pediatricians and allergists that they saw almost no peanut allergy in their population. Israeli mothers told us that peanut was one of the first weaning foods in infants' diets, often as early as four months of age. We investigated this, comparing the rates of peanut allergy in Israeli children and UK Jewish children who shared a similar ancestral background. Infants in Israel were fed considerable quantities of peanut from the age of four months, whereas in the United Kingdom infants avoided peanut in the first year of life. We found the rate of peanut allergy in UK schoolchildren was ten times higher than in their Israel counterparts.

We started to wonder whether the problem of increasing food allergies was caused in part by our attempts at prevention. On this basis we conducted the LEAP (Learning Early About Peanut) study, which was an interventional investigation looking at 640 babies randomized to either early consumption of peanut or avoidance of peanut in the first year of life. The study was conducted in children at high risk of peanut allergy (determined by the existence of a past history of eczema or egg allergy). The LEAP study showed that early consumption of peanut reduced the prevalence of peanut allergy by 80 percent. More recently, the LEAP-On study has shown that the effects are persistent, even once the children stopped consuming peanut regularly.

Moreover, the EAT (Enquiring About Tolerance) study, which investigated more than thirteen hundred children, showed that the introduction of wheat, dairy, egg, peanut, fish, and sesame from three months of age in normal, previously exclusively breast-fed infants, was associated with a two-thirds reduction in the rate of food allergies. The study findings were not as clear and dramatic as in LEAP. This reduction was seen only in the children who actually consumed those foods regularly at a young age and followed the study protocol. While one of the difficulties in the EAT study was successfully introducing multiple food allergens into infants' diets at a young age (many parents in the study were concerned about exposing their children to new foods, especially potentially allergy-causing ones), the EAT study nonetheless points the way toward the possibility of preventing all food allergies through early consumption of food. This study still needs to be replicated and strategies for early weaning developed, but Robin's book is an inspired and creative attempt to overcome some of these early weaning difficulties.

There now seems to be general consensus that early consumption of peanut in infants in the first year of life is recommended particularly for children at risk of developing allergies who have a family history of allergy or who have eczema themselves. While the question of whether eating multiple food allergens early in life will prevent all food allergies remains open to further confirmation, the balance of evidence is swinging toward early introduction of common food allergens (egg, wheat, peanut, fish, milk, sesame). Nevertheless, there is a lingering fear in the general medical and pediatric communities and among parents about introducing food allergens at an early age in children. While there is no doubt that babies who develop severe eczema in the first year of life may already have food allergies and require specialist advice before certain foods are introduced into their diets, there is no reason for other infants to avoid these foods beyond six months of age.

Robin is familiar with this fear. I remember meeting her more than five years ago when her then infant daughter first became my patient. She balked when I told her to give baby Clara eggs and nuts. And she was *not* going to leave my office until she understood the science behind my advice! I think she'd be the first to tell you that if I hadn't taken the time that day to help assuage her concerns, she might not have complied with my instructions. And Clara would likely still be suffering from life-threatening nut allergies.

Which is why I am so grateful that Robin, here, has taken the time to explain the science behind the new understanding of food allergies. As a reputable science writer and a former PhD candidate with a science degree from Columbia University, not to mention a mother of three, Robin analyzes the most recent studies and presents their findings in a way that all parents will be able to grasp.

Currently diet and nutrition books advising parents on how to wean infants adopt a very bland approach with emphasis on slow and delayed introduction of foods focusing initially on baby rice and pureed fruits and vegetables. Robin offers something far more exciting. She is passionate about introducing infants to healthful and delicious foods, especially potentially allergenic foods, based in large part on her own experience as a mother and also based on her understanding of recent research as a medical journalist. There is a gap in our knowledge about how to satisfy the palates of our infants and get them to enjoy a diverse and healthful diet, and Robin's book bridges that divide.

GIDEON LACK, MD,
Professor of Paediatric Allergy, King's College London;
Head of Clinical Academic Paediatric Allergy Service
for Guy's & St. Thomas' NHS Foundation Trust,
St. Thomas' Hospital, London

ALLERGY-FREE KIDS

Introduction

Around lunchtime one spring day, I sat Arthur, ten months old and my third child, in the grass outside my middle child's nursery school. Just four months earlier, Arthur would cry, sweat, and break out in hives whenever he touched cooked eggs. But I kept giving them to him, in small amounts on a daily basis, and on this day he squealed with delight and impatience when he saw I had packed him a hard-boiled egg.

Trisha Woodfire sat down beside me. She is lanky with the elongated arms and legs of a ballerina; she normally has an airy, unpredictable quality like a helium balloon just let go, but lately she seems weighted, steadied almost, by a perfectly globular pregnant belly.

I met Trisha, as so many moms meet, picking up our sons from the same nursery school. We'd chat politely, passing the time at the school gate, until we could see our sons' smiles again. But when I mentioned the topic of this book, Trisha became animated, curious and ready to share. Suddenly there was not enough time to talk, so we agreed to meet early one day so I could interview her formally about her experience with her oldest child's food allergies.

Every first-time parent has a lot of adjusting to do, many sleepless nights, and a lot of stress. But Trisha remembers three-year-old Henry's babyhood with breathless anxiety and darkness. He never slept more than twenty or thirty minutes at a time and seemed to be in constant agony. He was prone to projectile vomiting and had stools that smelled of "sickness, vinegar." Doctors and other medical professionals proved unhelpful.

"I was passed off as an overanxious mum," she told me. "But my instincts said, something is *wrong*."

Finally, Henry was diagnosed with dairy and soy allergies. Once these two allergens were removed from his diet, Henry was fine. He slept well and settled easily. But the dietician kept pushing her to "challenge" Henry with both dairy and soy by reintroducing small amounts and gradually increasing the dose until there was an adverse reaction.

"'We've got to see if he has outgrown it yet,' she would say," Trisha told me, shaking her head.

Trisha loathed doing the challenges. She would slowly work her way up the "milk ladder," which ranks the potency of the dairy protein in a particular food. She would start by giving Henry a fairly innocuous milk biscuit every day for four days and then move on to a pancake every day for four days and then some type of white sauce (over, say, lasagna) for four days until poor Henry had a reaction. She hated the cooking and the stringency of needing to keep the rest of his diet identical so she could know for sure it was the increase in dairy that was causing a reaction.

But most of all, she loathed making her kid sick. She went through it all the same, at the dietician's insistence, putting Henry through five dairy challenges and a similar number of soy challenges over the first two years of his life.

She remembers these years as ones of considerable stress, exhaustion, and ultimately, depression. But then, she said, continuing with a look of elation, "something changed in his body when he was two and a half, and I thought, he is better now."

Sure enough, the next challenge went swimmingly and Henry now has Greek yogurt for breakfast every morning and regularly has cooked milk and cheese. He also eats processed soy and has no reaction.

"I haven't yet tried cold milk from the fridge," she said, but they will get there. Of the allergy's disappearance, she says, "He just grew out of it."

When she says this, I can't help but wonder, did he really grow out of it, or did she accidentally desensitize him?

The conversation paused. I was not sure what to say in response. The experts I had been talking to recently would suspect the latter: By feeding Henry allergens early and often, Trisha helped Henry's immune system learn these were safe foods. Should I tell her?

In journalism classes, I was taught to stay mostly silent when conducting an interview. And my brief foray into psychological research (I ended up pursuing a degree in neuroscience instead), also taught me to stay mum in an interview. Do the asking, not the talking. The best info or quote always comes in the silences while the person tries to fill the dead air. As an interviewer, whether for journalism or academic research, I always tried to simply be a receptacle of information. Absorb, don't share.

To make things more confusing, the research I had my fingers on was *so* new. Some of it hadn't even been thoroughly digested yet by other scientists and researchers in the field. In academia, research that hasn't been properly vetted by the scientific community, should, well, be treated like it does not exist.

I resolved to keep my mouth shut.

Trisha filled the void of silence by patting her belly and we laughed about how "tidy" her pregnancy is so far. (She still looks like a ballerina but one who has swallowed a basketball.) As she told me she is expecting a girl, my thoughts tumbled on in private.

If her daughter exhibits similar problems, Trisha will surely try cutting out dairy and soy right away. But would she bother doing the food challenges again? Would she go back to the same dietician, who kept harping on her? Would she set herself up for a repeat scenario of stress and darkness? Or would she just wait a couple years, avoiding allergens, with the possibly misguided understanding that eventually her daughter would "just grow out of it"?

Projecting myself into Trisha's future with a baby and a preschooler to keep tabs on, I imagined her deciding not to torture her daughter with food challenges, the way she did her son. (Don't worry, as we'll see, there is a way to introduce allergens without torture!) Skipping the food challenges would save her whole household from the stress of a sick, sleepless baby. She could just wait, I imagined her thinking, until her daughter "outgrew it."

But *would* her daughter grow out of it if she wasn't regularly exposed to small amounts of milk the way her brother was? The majority of kids do outgrow dairy and soy allergies. But many carry the allergy into adulthood, and for some it can become life threatening.

Not only does the baby in Trisha's tummy have an increased risk of food allergies due to her brother's condition, she also has a family history of serious autoimmune disorders. Autoimmune diseases and allergies are both on the rise for unexplained, presumably "modern" reasons. It is unclear whether one is a risk factor for the other, but it seems that the so-called modern lifestyle, which has its many perks, including relatively low rates of infectious diseases, is also likely having various effects on the immune systems of many people. In my own family, I have two young cousins with type 1 diabetes, and my brother and I have celiac disease, an autoimmune disorder where gluten damages the small intestine. I was diagnosed at nineteen, confirmed later by blood test, after my weight dropped below ninety pounds on my five-foot six-inch frame. Perhaps counterintuitively, after cutting out bread, cakes, pasta, and all other gluten-containing products, I returned to a normal weight. (This was in the 1990s, before all the yummy gluten-free substitutes became as widely available as they are today.) My husband's family also has various autoimmune disorders.

In Trisha's family, her sister suffers from multiple sclerosis, and Trisha herself, when she was twenty-four, had a bout of facial weakness and double vision that lasted for six weeks. She was diagnosed with a type of "temporary" multiple sclerosis, she said. Last, but not least, of all, it is looking like Trisha's husband may have celiac disease.

As Trisha explained the various illnesses in her family, my resolve began to weaken. If the means existed to protect her baby from just one of many possible health problems, she surely deserved to know. Of course, it is impossible to say whether Trisha cured Henry or he simply outgrew it. We will never know. But with her daughter, wouldn't she prefer to be safe than sorry?

I wrestled with myself. Should I keep quiet? Or should I, carefully, tell her everything I know? Should I respect her own intelligence and knowledge of her own children to take the information and do the best she could with it?

Two weeks earlier, I interviewed Pippa George in the same village green, a large square field that is the heart of our tiny English village. (We are originally from New York but moved to London when our oldest was a newborn and then set out for the English countryside when I became pregnant with our second child.) Pippa has blond, straight, shoulder-length hair; a dazzling smile; and a youthful, supremely kind persona. She brought Oliver, eighteen months old, with her. Oliver is blond like his mother and an independent chap; he heads off toward the road, again and again, as if he has a magnetic draw to cars. (Fortunately they are nearly all parked cars in this quiet nook.) She chases him, each time laughing into the sunshine and swinging him, like a bushel of hay, back over to where we are talking about her older son, Ben, who is four.

When Ben was Oliver's age, he nearly died after coming in contact with a cashew. Pippa's household, understandably, has been completely nut-free ever since. His nursery carries an EpiPen for him and the school asks all other parents to strictly avoid putting nut products in packed lunches on the days he attends.

His little brother, Oliver, has not yet had any allergic reactions, but as a baby he had eczema, which is considered a warning sign of coming food allergies. If Oliver had my kids' doctor, he would have been introduced to nuts in early infancy, almost as a vaccination against developing allergies. But after his big brother's experiences, Oliver has never come in contact with a nut or nut butter of any kind.

I understand the logic behind Pippa's choices. She has made them out of love and fear. They are the same ones I would have made for my kids if I hadn't been so lucky to be referred to a doctor conducting cutting-edge research. Research that suggests we can protect most kids from food allergies, simply by introducing allergens early and often.

Should I say something?

Pippa put Oliver in a swing and said, wincing, "I read this article about giving small amounts [of allergens], but I am so scared." I sympathized. And folded. I told her what I know—and just as important—what I don't. I trusted her to use the information with intelligence and reserve, and to seek the guidance of a good doctor.

And here I was again, in the same grass, listening to another mom, wondering if I should talk. I looked at Trisha's protruding belly, sighed, and let the floodgates open. I talked about not only the published studies but also the ones that are in progress. I told her where the research is heading. I told her that all her hard work, persevering through so many food challenges, may actually be the reason Henry is now allergy-free.

Her eyes opened wide. And then she smiled, glimmering with wonder and a slice of pride. Perhaps it wasn't all for naught.

Why I Wrote This Book

....

The above was over a year ago. The studies I was watching develop then have all been vetted and published, some with straightforward findings and others with more complicated messages. The overarching philosophy—*feed kids allergens, early and often*—is now being grasped by many major members of the medical community and is particularly well regarded when it comes to peanut allergy. Research is continuing as you read. And many questions remain: What is the optimal amount, and form, of each allergen for conferring protection from an allergy? Will protecting from food allergy help protect from environmental allergies and asthma? What is the age range of the critical window for each food allergen and why do they differ? Will early exposure protect kids from all food allergies, even ones that haven't been adequately studied yet, such as kiwi, soy, and citrus fruits? Are there unintended consequences to early exposure to

....

**Especially if your baby has dry skin,
eczema, a family history of food allergies,
or other signs that food allergies may
already be present, have him tested before
introducing food allergens.**

....

allergens that could have an adverse health effect? (One of the most significant worries was that early exposure would lead to premature weaning, but research has shown it does not shorten breast-feeding duration.)

Furthermore, while we now have some significant insights into how we might prevent food allergies, overcoming existing allergies is still very tricky. Desensitization protocols for most allergens currently need to be tailored to the individual and overseen by a medical professional. And unfortunately, they may not work for every allergy sufferer.

In other words, we don't have all the answers yet. The information is going to keep coming out and the advice is likely to be tweaked as we go forward. (Watch this book's page on my website, RobinNixonPompa.com, for updates.) But I believe the tip of an iceberg of understanding has been found. As the years progress, I expect we will only learn more and more about the benefits of exposing the infant immune system to potential allergens.

Perhaps I should have waited until every detail was ironed out to write this book. I did think about it. I am a sleep-deprived, full-time mother of three children under five years old. Postponing this book had serious appeal!

But then I thought of Oliver, and Trisha's unborn daughter, and the hundreds of thousands of little ones who were about to pass out of the presumed critical window during which their allergy could have been prevented. I thought of the stress and fear many families live with every day, how it hampers their lives, restricting and prohibiting simple joys like spontaneously stopping for a bite at a diner or taking road trips, where all food will be prepared by others; arranging first-time playdates, which will now entail a lengthy explanation of food rules; and attending birthday parties and sleepovers, for which separately packaged food may be required. I thought of the child's fear, knowing that food—something that should rightly be a source of pleasure and contentment—has the capacity to kill her, suddenly and painfully. And of course I thought of the few, but still too many, children who will never reach adulthood, despite the years of painstaking diligence over their every bite. I thought of the pain of parents who have lost their child to anaphylactic shock. When I would think about all of this, I couldn't keep my mouth shut—or my hands off my computer. Parents deserve to know that new scientific findings are starting to change medical recommendations, from advice to avoid allergens to encouragement to embrace them.

*   *   *

The logic used to be, let's wait for the immune system to be mature enough, or for the child to be old enough to express discomfort, before introducing potentially trouble-making allergens. *But now studies suggest that for most babies allergens are safe. And avoiding them may make food allergies more likely.*

Many scientists are proposing that the immune system has a critical window in which it can be taught that allergens are not dangerous. This window likely starts slowly closing between four and six months of age and is mostly, although not completely, shut by late childhood, possibly as early as five years old. But some researchers hypothesize that for most kids it can be propped permanently open by repeated exposure to food allergens over the first five years of life.

If you can get your kids to eat them.

And this is the rub: Many kids do not like the taste of common allergens, so how do we get our kids to swallow them—especially without gagging, tears, or coercion?

With a bit of perseverance, we can have our (allergen-filled) cake and eat it, too. I've lived it. All three of my children have suffered from food allergies, with reactions ranging from irritating to potentially life threatening, and we are now, most likely due to the advice and recipes in this book, an allergy-free household. I can't tell you the daily relief it has given our family to not have to worry about what our children eat outside of the house. Then again, if you have a child with a food allergy, I don't need to tell you. You know. It is much more than a nuisance; it is a nagging fear that saturates all corners of your life.

I do sometimes struggle with protecting our new freedom from food fear. To keep the allergies from returning or new ones from developing, I've been advised to keep my kids eating all major allergens on a twice-weekly basis. This can be hard work and I have often been met with resistance from my children. I've tried a variety of tactics, employing both psychological tricks and recipe tweaks, to help make sure my kids eat their allergens and thus stay allergy-free. I've put my best strategies into this book, aiming to relieve the stress not only of allergies but also of the work of allergy prevention and to bring joy back to family meals.

To put the growing problem of food allergies in context, chapter 1 covers the prevailing theories on why allergies are sky-rocketing worldwide and the science that is being used to try to untangle this mystery. Chapter 2 describes the medical research that enabled doctors to discover that many food allergies can be prevented and, in some cases, that an allergy sufferer can be helped to become largely desensitized to foods that previously caused adverse reactions.

Chapter 3 gives overall advice for preventing allergy development in children and babies. It discusses the various challenges in feeding children from infancy to age five and the complications that can arise when you are feeding more than one child, each with their own needs and tastes. The advice in this chapter has been influenced by the work of nutritionists, psychologists, pediatricians, and registered dieticians, but *it is not meant to be a comprehensive guide to feeding and nutrition.* Rather, it gives tips and strategies for helping your child eat the dose of allergen she needs to be safe.

I've grouped these strategies according to age. Feeding an infant is obviously much different from feeding a preschooler, but even the changes that happen between four and seven months old, or between fifteen and twenty-four months, can be significant. Our parents said it and their parents said it: Kids grow up so fast. This is particularly true in the first five years when the brain nearly quadruples in size and the rate of change in physical and mental abilities dwarfs that of any other time in life. *And it is these first five years that doctors think is likely the most important time for teaching the immune system that all foods are safe.*

Please don't take the age categories in this book as rigid and worry if your child doesn't, say, grab for your spoon yet. Imagine the age categories more as groupings that blur and overlap one another; every child is different, and if what works for most doesn't work for yours, it is not a statement of failure but rather one of individuality. Similarly, if tricks that helped your six-month-old still work at eighteen months, fantastic! *If it ain't broke . . .* Chapter 3 also discusses the difficulties that can arise when an allergic child gains a sibling; you will want to prevent allergy development in the baby by exposing him to all major allergens, while simultaneously keeping the older, already-allergic child safe.

Chapter 4 gives the specifics of strategies for allergy prevention, explaining the "doses" of each allergen that are currently hypothesized to be protective and providing a brief discussion of how to handle worries about certain food allergens, like soy and kiwi, that haven't been expressly studied yet.

Chapter 5 is devoted to recipes that may help prevent common food allergies. These have been roughly divided by allergen; there is a section each for eggs, nuts, sesame, dairy, wheat, and fish. For your convenience, however, many of the recipes target two, three, or eight allergies at once. There is a list of these powerhouse recipes and meal ideas on page 99.

Please read about each allergen in chapter 4 before delving into the cooking. Each allergen has its own quirks and potential complications in serving a baby or toddler.

An important note about using this book: Every year that goes by—and most of the studies take several years to complete—in which parents are avoiding allergens and kids are passing out of the critical window for prevention means thousands more people are sentenced to a lifetime of being worried that something on their plate may kill them. With this sense of urgency in mind, while simultaneously remembering that we have loads left to learn, this book gives the best advice based on what we know *now*—always erring on the side of caution and safety.

Please use this book in conjunction with the advice of a pediatrician or allergist—especially if your child is considered at high risk of developing an allergy. Babies and children with eczema, allergic siblings, or parents with eczema or any food or environmental allergies are considered at high risk for developing a food allergy.

Science is a quickly changing field and your allergist may know of new ways to treat your little one. Also, while the vast majority of children can be helped with the advice in this book, some may have more complicated problems. *If you are concerned, or see troublesome signs such as rough skin or hives, have her evaluated by a doctor.* I wish I had known this. All three of my babies had slightly dry skin, but I thought nothing of it the first time. We didn't have my oldest tested for allergies until after going through a quite scary allergic event. A doctor later explained to me that babies should have smooth, soft skin; if not, it can be a cause for concern.

As for the recipes, each aims to be nutritious, kid friendly, and allergy fighting. The vast majority are also easy to make, convenient to serve, and even freezable. After all, they are primarily for parents of very young children and babies—people who never have enough hands, let alone time. The best tactic, I find, is to choose some recipe that works for your little one, make lots on that one Sunday you have free, and freeze enough for daily feeding the rest of the month. Or maybe it is easier in your household to declare two days a week allergy-fighting days and give your child his doses then. Either way is fine as long as the allergens are consumed in the recommended weekly doses over at least two days.

As I was writing this book, I had three kids under age five, so each recipe was developed with little ones underfoot, resting on my hip, or usually both. I gave the kids official titles as my helpers, depending on the tasks or recipe of the day: sous-chef, taste checker, sorter, even illustrator. While the older two often got involved in the stirring and measuring, the preferred duties by far were pushing the buttons on the food processor, unwrapping and breaking up baking chocolate (probably because the odds were good that I'd offer them a piece), and taste-testing the finished products. The last "job" was done with a solemnity that never failed to make me laugh, even if the verdicts were rarely nuanced. I would get either "It's good, Mama!" or "I don't really like it." If all three said the latter, I'd scratch the recipe and try again. But if at least two declared it "yummy scrummy, more please," I'd make it again—and jot it down for you and yours to try. I hope you have as much fun making the recipes in this book as my kids and I did developing them.

As for ideas for the recipes, nineteen came directly from the Enquiring About Tolerance (EAT) study, which is discussed in detail in chapter 2. Briefly, in the per-protocol analysis of this three-year study of over thirteen hundred healthy newborns, babies who had early, regular exposure to allergens were 67 percent less likely to have developed a food allergy by toddlerhood. It also showed that early exposure is safe; there was not one case of an anaphylactic reaction in the entire study.

To help parents expose their babies to allergens regularly, the EAT study researchers gave participants a handbook that included recipes, many of which combine allergens into a single dish, to make feeding kids allergens early and often an easy, painless task. The researchers involved in this study gave these recipes to me, to share with you.

The remaining recipes involved searching blogs, product websites, and cookbooks. I often combined ideas and tried to simplify techniques for a busy family. One of my favorite tricks is to cook something in an oven that you could just as well do on a stovetop. At least in my house, the fifteen minutes before dinner can be hectic and, with falling blood sugar, grumpy. Whenever I can, I have dinner preparing itself in the oven, so I can have my hands free to comfort a tearful toddler or read to an impatient preschooler. I have also prioritized recipes that are easy to make with one hand and that can be made in bulk and frozen for easy meals later in the month.

One more note, for my fellow health-conscious parents: I am not a dietician and none of the advice in this book should be taken as medical advice on childhood nutrition. That said, in general, when feeding a child, I think hiding nutrients misses the point. I have found eating handfuls of greens myself to be the best strategy for sharing my love of vegetables with my children, as opposed to trying to sneak them in via a beet brownie. (While I've never known a brownie to be refused, kale-chip night in our house is an avidly anticipated weekly event.)

But when it comes to allergens, my philosophy changes. It is not about teaching healthful-eating principles—for example, that vegetables should be a substantial part of every meal—but rather about "dosing" my children's immune system, guiding its development, so that my kids might be less likely to have their food allergies return, more likely to develop healthful relationships with food, and more likely to *fearlessly* eat a wide variety of foods. So when preparing allergens, I am happy to add a bit extra sugar, butter, or starch and to disguise them as something more palatable: cookies, burgers, even funny woodland animals.

I content myself with the fact that my kids are overall healthful eaters: Grant, my two-year-old, is currently obsessed with raw red bell peppers; Arthur, ten months, squeals over roasted broccoli; and four-year-old Clara's favorite, if asked, is cottage cheese or, maybe, strawberries. So when it comes time for the daily allergen treat, if "a little sugar makes the medicine go down," well, truly, isn't that the most delightful way—for all of us? (And don't worry, I really mean just a *little* sugar.)

Because what I *really* don't want is for the stress over allergies to become a stress about eating. I want family mealtimes to be ones of celebration ("Look at all the good food! Aren't we lucky!"), not ones of struggle, negotiation, or bribery ("If you eat your egg, you can have a Popsicle."). That said, in the case of allergies, if it takes negotiations and bribes to get the medicine down, so be it. It is for the best.

But my primary hope is that every family can avoid struggle. Which is why I wrote this book.

IN AN ALLERGY-FREE NUTSHELL

1. Avoiding allergens could make food allergies more likely.

2. The immune system may have a critical window, within which it can be most easily taught that all foods are safe.

3. This critical window is best seized from three to five months old through toddlerhood.

4. There may be ways to address food allergies in later childhood; research is ongoing.

5. While allergens are now considered safe for most infants, please use this book in conjunction with the advice of a pediatrician or allergist if your child has dry skin or a family history of allergies.

6. To have a possible protective effect, allergens need to be given both early and often. Intermittent exposure is not enough.

7. Some kids will develop food allergies no matter how well protected.

Chapter 1

The Problem

I'll be the first to say it: Having a kid with a food allergy sucks. So let's steer clear of it (the allergy, not the kid).

Research is starting to suggest a simple way that many parents can prevent a lifetime of EpiPen touting, label reading, and waiter quizzing. (That said, some kids may become food allergic no matter how well we try to protect them.)

Feed your kid allergens early, carefully, and often.

This strategy turns previous recommendations on their heads. At the turn of the century, parents were advised to avoid major food allergens, such as wheat, nut, egg, soy, dairy, fish, and shellfish, for their child's first few years of life. But now studies show that avoidance is likely among the very things contributing to the allergy epidemic.

Instead of avoiding allergens, most of us should be sneaking them into our kids' snacks, sandwiches, even their sippy cups. Embracing allergens could turn them from potential foes to friends.

Today, an estimated 6 to 8 percent of children and one in ten preschool children in developed countries, such as the United States, the United Kingdom, and Australia, have a clinically diagnosed food allergy, leaving millions of parents wielding EpiPens, scouring food packages at birthday parties, and panicking that someone may offer their child a snack. Every three minutes a food allergy sends someone to an emergency room, according to the *Journal of Allergy and Clinical Immunology*. That is roughly two hundred thousand emergency visits per year. Up to one-third of these reactions are ones of anaphylaxis, in which the immune system launches an attack on the body that can be fatal if not arrested within the first ten to twenty minutes by an adrenaline injection via an EpiPen.

Previous generations did not have this worry. Food allergies among children are on a startling rise. They rose 50 percent between 1997 and 2011, according to the Centers for Disease Control and Prevention. And the rate of increase may be accelerating. A 2015 study by the European Academy of Allergy and Clinical Immunology found that the prevalence of food allergy had doubled within the previous decade and the number of hospitalizations for severe allergic reactions had increased sevenfold.

Anaphylaxis is not the only concern. Food allergies have been associated with malnutrition and increased psychological issues, due to the stress and possible social isolation. They are also considered only one step of the "atopic march." First comes eczema in infancy, allergies in toddlerhood, and then asthma in kindergarten.

My daughter Clara, as an infant, swelled into a bawling tomato the first time I fed her scrambled eggs. Worried that her airways would constrict, we called emergency services. It was one of the scariest moments of my life—and from what I hear on the playground and at school pickup, it is an experience that has become shockingly commonplace. Today, nearly six million kids in the United States and one million in the United Kingdom have food allergies.

Skin-prick and blood testing found that in addition to Clara's egg allergy, she had life-threatening nut allergies. (Egg allergy is actually a risk factor for nut allergies.) We were told she'd have to be extremely careful for the rest of her life. We put an EpiPen in every purse and bag, scoured food labels, scrupulously kept most nuts out of the house and warned friends, family, babysitters, and nursery teachers, repeatedly, and especially before going to their houses, that our precious toddler was likely to die on their floor if they did not keep nuts—and nut products like Nutella, marzipan, granola, pesto, many cakes, chocolates, and cookies—out of her reach. It did not make us very popular, and I worried all the stress would lead to psychological feeding and eating issues. But it was worth Clara's safety.

Fortunately, our approach to Clara's allergies did not stop with simple avoidance. In addition to the antihistamines and EpiPen prescriptions, our allergist, medical researcher Dr. Gideon Lack, also had some unusual advice on how to feed Clara.

Dear reader, he said to give her a daily dose of nuts and eggs! Okay, not the nuts she was allergic to (almond, cashew, pistachio, macadamia, Brazil, and hazelnut) but the types of nut that had been deemed safe by skin prick and blood tests (pine nut, peanut, pecan, and walnut). And we were to give her one-twentieth of an egg.

I must have looked at him bug eyed when he said this, as I imagined carefully measuring and dissecting an omelet and coaxing a tiny spoonful down my daughter's throat. No, he shook his head as if he had seen my expression on the face of one mother too many. We were to make a cake using only one egg and give her one-twentieth of it. Every day. After a month or so, we were to put two eggs in the cake and then three. A daily slice of cake on doctor's orders? Clara was in heaven.

We followed his instructions to the letter, and today, at four years old, Clara no longer has food allergies. While, true, the egg allergy may have resolved itself eventually no matter, as many kids grow out of egg allergy, the eggy cake slices she ate likely accelerated this resolution significantly. As for her multiple nut allergies, we were originally told that they would be with her for life since it is unusual for kids to "outgrow" allergies to nuts. It is not conclusively known, but the daily exposure to her four safe nuts may have helped resolve these other six allergies by teaching her immune system that nuts aren't bad after all. When both her brothers, as infants, had visible reactions to eggs, we turned again to what we had learned from Dr. Lack. My youngest also regularly broke out in hives after consuming sesame, both whole sesame seeds and the ground form found in hummus, but the reactions have since subsided. (Sesame allergy is potentially very dangerous; approach a doctor, if you suspect your child is allergic to sesame or any other seed or nut.) Today, with three young children, our house is allergy-free.

Historical Approach?

While the strategy of small regular doses has revolutionized the face of food allergy prevention and treatment, the concept isn't that new to medicine or general biology. Born in 135 BCE, King Mithridates VI is said to have used a similar approach to avoid being poisoned by his mother. Unable to protect himself externally from her wily ways (she likely poisoned his father), he built up internal resistance by gradually ingesting larger and larger quantities of poisons until he was immune. Mithridatism, as the strategy is still sometimes called, has been used many times in popular culture, perhaps most memorably in the movie *The Princess Bride* where, after psychological second and triple guessing, we find that not one but both cups set before the hero are laced with poison— only Wesley, the trickster and other drinker, has acquired immunity to the poison by ingesting small graduated amounts.

In Austria, the legendary "arsenic eaters of Styria" are said to have done much the same thing. These peasants would start with a tiny amount of poison and gradually build up the amount of arsenic they ate over the course of several weeks until they were ingesting quantities that would kill most people, according to an 1869 issue of *Scientific American*. The waxing and waning of the moon was apparently used to guide the graduated increase and then decrease of ingestion. Arsenic eaters, described in the report as "generally strong and healthy persons, courageous, pugnacious, and of strong sexual dispositions," reported that their main motivation for taking arsenic was to increase strength and health!

These examples are particularly pertinent in the case of food allergy as the allergic body, albeit erroneously, reacts to allergens *as if* they are poison. And it is this reaction, rather than the food itself, that ends up being the killer. The immune system goes into overdrive, attacking the perceived invader, and in the worst cases, a series of chemical miscommunications and feedback loops, called anaphylaxis, cause airways to constrict and the lungs or heart to collapse. The allergy sufferer becomes an innocent casualty of an imagined war.

> **We need to help the immune system
> learn that foods are safe.**

These responses can be avoided by "educating" the immune system to correctly recognize innocuous substances. Such training starts with minute amounts of the allergen or poison, and by increasing the amount gradually over a period of time, immunity may be achieved to nearly all allergens (but not all poisons!). The immunity is often temporary, however. If the immune system is given time to "forget" the training, over a course of discontinued exposure, a full, fatal response can result from a previously safe dose.

Today, such training is usually called oral immunotherapy. Immunotherapy is just that: therapy for the immune system, correcting any erroneous, destructive tendencies and treating it, carefully and gently, by gradually giving it larger and larger doses of allergens, until it is able to appropriately recognize friend from foe on its own.

Immunotherapy has long been successful in treating other types of allergies, such as severe hay fever and allergies to bee and wasp stings. An allergen dose can be given by injection or "sublingually" via a tablet or drop placed under the tongue. Or orally, which is better known as eating.

Clinically speaking, immunotherapy is considered successful when the immune system starts producing certain regulatory cells that stop the production of immunoglobulin E (IgE), the sometimes "bad guy" largely responsible for misidentifying and attacking innocuous allergens, giving rise to adverse allergic reactions. Immunotherapy puts IgE in its place.

In addition to treating allergies, oral immunotherapy is being explored by scientists in the United States and Germany as a possible way to prevent type 1 diabetes. While diabetes is not an allergy, it shares one commonality: an immune system gone haywire. Instead of the immune system's mistaking some stray peanut as a poison (as happens with peanut allergy), a diabetic's immune system thinks insulin-producing pancreatic cells are poison. Both involve a misguided war launched by the immune system, the end game being anaphylaxis in peanut allergy and destroyed pancreatic cells in diabetes. It is very interesting that they might both be prevented with the same treatment: oral introduction of the offending substance at a predisease stage. While the research on the prevention of type 1 diabetes needs further development, the research on the prevention of food allergies is now relatively well substantiated.

In a sense, the strategy rests on the same logic as vaccination, which is largely considered the most lifesaving advance of medical history. While, true, vaccinations are usually targeting infectious diseases, and rarely require more than one or two doses, they work by "educating" the immune system with minute quantities of the offending substance.

Increasingly, vaccinations are being used for respiratory allergies (think pollen, dust). And in the future, there may be vaccinations against food allergies. At least one trial study using a vaccine against fish allergies in Europe is showing promise, according to scientists writing in *Gastroenterology*.

But a spoonful of allergen puree at three months old may be just as good.

Clues to the Cause

The grade school Clara attends, like many schools these days, has strict rules against the quintessential childhood sandwich: the PB&J. For weeks, this was my biggest hurdle in getting Clara excited about school. (They start at age four in the United Kingdom.) Clara *loves* her nut butter and jam sandwiches; if going to school meant she could no longer have them for lunch, *perhaps school isn't such a good idea, Mama?* I was also worried; I'd need to find another way to make sure Clara was getting enough nut exposure to keep her allergies at bay.

It wasn't long until I met one of the mothers whose kid was responsible for the no PB&J stress in my household. Harsha, a sunny South African, has a lovely laugh and a warm, open demeanor. We fell into chatting at school pickups; she has a baby girl a couple months younger than Arthur, in addition to Deelan, who is seven years old and allergic to nuts, shellfish, coconut, grass, cats, and pollen.

Harsha and her sister grew up with allergies, which she says was unusual. "Allergies are less common in South Africa; my sister and I were an anomaly," she said, waving her hand, as if to imply I should discount her own family's experiences. "The kids seem bigger, sturdier, there than here [in England]," she added, flexing the muscles in her arms imitating the kids in South Africa.

Due to her own experience with allergies, and worried about Deelan's eczema, Harsha carefully followed the UK government's advice, as prescribed by her pediatrician, and avoided all major allergens throughout his infancy and toddlerhood. She breast-fed exclusively for the first four months and then began supplementing with formula. She introduced solids extremely slowly, not giving him more than a few spoonfuls until he was at least eight months old.

Then, when he was eighteen months old, Deelan tried a prawn and broke out in hives all over his body. A few months later, he had a sauce in a restaurant with cashew in it. He again broke out in hives. Familiar with allergies, Harsha gave him a half dose of an antihistamine in each case. They now keep both antihistamines and an EpiPen readily available.

After these experiences, Harsha has made sure Deelan strictly avoids all nuts and shellfish. When he turned four years old and would be starting school soon, she petitioned the public health system and had him properly tested for allergies.

The skin-prick testing turned out to be quite traumatizing for Deelan. His whole arm swelled into an itchy red sore. He doesn't want to ever *ever* go back to the hospital for subsequent testing. So to be safe, Harsha just makes sure Deelan continues to strictly avoid all nuts and shellfish.

Deelan also has wheat intolerance, which she hopes he'll grow out of, as it is the food issue that troubles him most socially. "They don't really serve shellfish and nuts at birthday parties," Harsha pointed out. "But cake . . ." Her voice trailed off as she imagined his regular deprivation.

As it is, he carries with him a specially prepared box of food just for him to birthday parties and other major social occasions. When the school has afternoon bake sales, and the other kids swarm around the tables begging their mothers for coins to buy chocolate cupcakes, he shrugs with a sigh and walks off toward home.

Although she is aware of the social strain Deelan's allergies can cause, Harsha seems mostly unconcerned about his physical health. "He has known to ask, since he was very small, what is in anything he is handed to eat."

She is more fretful over her infant daughter, whose allergies remain unknown. After feeding Liana some "baby's first porridge" concoction and watching her break out in hives around her mouth, Harsha is now worried about milk and soy. When she tried to introduce formula milk to Liana, again there were hives. And eczema has been a problem basically since birth.

I told Harsha about my experience and gave her Dr. Lack's contact information. She listened politely about my introduction of allergenic foods to Arthur, but I sensed she was too scared, and scarred from her experiences with Deelan, to introduce any major allergens beyond cow's milk to *her* new baby.

Deelan and Liana have plenty of company. At least two children in every class of twenty to twenty-four kids at Clara's small school have a prominent food allergy or intolerance. I have never been asked about the topic of this book and not been given a personal story in return, usually about their own child or that of a friend or sibling. The statistic claiming that nearly 8 percent of kids have some form of food allergy is hardly surprising to anyone, especially the teachers and other personnel, at school drop-off.

On the Rise

This prevalence is a new development. Over the last couple decades, researchers have watched in bafflement over the rise in allergies and asthma. While they are thought to be primarily genetic conditions, the recent rise has been too steep to be explained by heredity alone. When I was chatting with Dr. James Baker, the chief medical officer of Food Allergy Research and

Education, he mentioned that he believes the rise in allergies in modern times has been caused by "a fundamental change in the human immune system."

It must be. Because food allergies do not make evolutionary sense. Hunters and gatherers who dropped dead after tasting a seed, nut, or egg, would rarely have lived long enough to reproduce. That is, natural selection would have, *must have*, selected against food allergies. Therefore, their current rise must be the result of recent changes in our environments and/or lifestyles, scientists point out, likely due to an epigenetic process that has sped up the resulting changes in our bodies. Epigenetics is an emerging field studying how our environments and lifestyles can change our genes, even in the germ line, meaning they are inheritable. A population can be more quickly changed through this route than through classical natural selection.

But just which environmental or lifestyle changes are responsible for the rise in food allergies, nobody knows.

Peanut allergy has been studied most extensively, perhaps because it is deemed the worst allergy to have. Peanuts and tree nuts are considered the most fatal allergies, according to the American Academy of Allergy, Asthma and Immunology, killing 150 to 200 people a year just in the United States. And while kids often grow out of egg and dairy allergies (albeit more slowly these days), nut allergies usually stick around for life. This makes nut allergy a bit simpler to study in large populations.

When looking across the globe, researchers first saw a marked difference in the amount of peanut allergy in developed countries such as England and the United States when compared to poorer nations in Africa and Asia. While the data are hard to collect precisely due to different reporting standards, richer countries, on average, have been thought to have roughly ten times more peanut allergy than poorer countries. (That said, developing countries seem to be catching up as they modernize, according to the World Allergy Organization.)

Theories run amok on why this would be the case: Pollution, fast food, prenatal supplements, decline in breast-feeding, increases in caesarean section, improved sanitation, lack of sunshine, exposure to tobacco smoke, and other ideas have had differing levels of support. Let's explore the ones with the most compelling evidence.

You Are My Sunshine, My *Only* Sunshine

According to one popular theory, the rise in all food allergies is being caused by vitamin D deficiency, a growing problem in developed countries due to our indoor lifestyles and the resulting lack of exposure to sunlight. Some researchers posit that the decrease in vitamin D levels across many populations has been in lockstep with the rise in food allergies.

Further correlational data lend support to the theory. Allergy rates increase as you move farther from the equator, even after adjusting for physician density and socioeconomic status. (This latitude trend is also seen for multiple sclerosis, schizophrenia, and Parkinson's, three other conditions for which the role of vitamin D is currently being examined.) A study in Boston, which sounds like astrology but is actually hard science, found that patients visiting a hospital due to food allergies were more likely to have an autumn or winter birthday. It seems that babies born in autumn or winter, when opportunities for sun exposure are low, are more likely to develop severe allergies than those born in the sunny summer months. (My babies don't fit; they were all born in the summer—but their infancies were spent in England and I am not sure England has a sun.)

In the United States, a study found that in the northernmost states, eight to twelve EpiPens were prescribed for every one thousand people, whereas in southern states, only three EpiPens per one thousand people were being prescribed. Multiple variables, such as density of doctors and socioeconomic status, were used to analyze the data, but nothing better explained the gradient than simple latitude. It was also found that in populations with a high incidence of skin cancer, EpiPen prescriptions were low and vice versa, giving further support to the theory that the north/south differences in allergy rates in the United States are due to sun exposure.

Similarly, a study undertaken in Australia, "down under" the equator, showed that kids growing up in the south, where there is less sunshine, were six times more likely to have a peanut allergy and twice as likely to have an egg allergy in comparison to kids of comparable socioeconomic status growing up in the northern part of the country. In 2013, the *Journal of Allergy and Clinical Immunology* published results from a study in which blood samples were taken from over five thousand babies. Researchers found that those who had low vitamin D levels were three times as likely to have food allergies.

While vitamin D deficiency may be contributing to the rise in food allergies, moderate sunlight, rather than supplements, may be the best response.

Mechanistic data supporting the role of vitamin D in immune system development are widely available. Receptors for vitamin D are widespread in the immune system, and vitamin D could influence both the onset and the resolution of food allergies through a variety of immunological pathways, according to researchers writing in *Food Allergy: Adverse Reactions to Foods and Food Additives*.

In particular, vitamin D supports the proper functioning of T cells—largely considered the immune system's infantry. Lack of vitamin D from sunlight during infancy and even during the mother's pregnancy could be causing dissension among the ranks, resulting in random erroneous strikes and painful friendly fire, giving rise to eczema, allergies, and various auto-immune diseases.

Unfortunately, the problem isn't so simple that vitamin supplementation is a straightforward answer. In already allergic children, the immune system has developed too far down the wrong path to be corrected by a dose of vitamin D. And for healthy infants, several studies have shown that vitamin D supplementation may actually increase the risk of food allergy. Furthermore, too much vitamin D via overeager supplementation can lead to other problems, such as nausea, confusion, abnormal heart rhythm, and kidney stones. Research is still being gathered, but it may be better to fight vitamin D deficiency by getting moderate sunshine rather than through supplementation.

The World Is Too Clean

The so-called hygiene hypothesis claims that the developed world's overly clean environments have given rise to allergies and autoimmune conditions. I am tempted to use this theory to put a positive spin on my hatred of housework—as in *my* kids couldn't possibly be victims of a too-clean environment, as our home, most of the time, best resembles a pigsty. However, despite its catchy name and the way the theory is usually reported in mainstream media—"Eating off the Floor: How Clean Living Is Bad for You" ran one 2012 headline in a guest blog on the *Scientific American* website—the hygiene hypothesis is not a license to stop scrubbing dishes or bathrooms. (Bummer, I know.) The theory is best understood as going beyond our immediate households, reflecting the cleanliness provided by improved sanitation, cleaner water, less contaminated food, and so on, which has drastically reduced infectious diseases and improved life spans.

These are obvious benefits, but there may be some downsides, too. Scientists have found that when mice are raised in a sterile environment, they tend to have dysfunctional immune systems and are prone to allergies, as explained by Jerome Groopman writing in the *New Yorker*. "It is possible that we are doing the same thing to ourselves," he suggests.

The immune system, scientists hypothesize, has to be challenged while young in order to develop properly. In a spotless world, where there are few pathogenic challenges, the idle immune system becomes paranoid and starts causing mischief, believing every stray particle or peanut to be poison.

The analogy is extrapolated from what we know about the visual system. While, admittedly, the visual system is in many ways different from the immune system, both have a significant development period that happens after birth. Using methods that would likely be considered cruel by today's standards, experiments conducted in the 1960s and 1970s, where the eyes of kittens were temporarily sutured shut, helped scientists discover that the visual system has a "critical period" during the first weeks of life. If kittens do not receive proper visual stimulation during this period, the visual system fails to develop properly. Born normal, kittens deprived of light are rendered effectively blind.

Similarly, researchers have proposed there may be a critical period for the infant immune system. If it is not adequately stimulated—by pathogens, diverse foods, and so forth—it will begin stumbling along, and be knocked over by things it should have "seen" clearly.

Falling under the hygiene hypothesis's umbrella is the old friends theory. This theory posits that our contact with "good" microbes has become insufficient, not only due to our necessary efforts to curb infectious disease but also due to our modern tendency to spend little time actually interacting with plants, animals, and "nature" on the whole. While we humans like to think of ourselves as solitary satellites operating above the fray of the larger, older world, growing research suggests "old friend" microbes are not only necessary for good digestion (think probiotics) but also for the proper development and functioning of our immune systems.

Providing supporting evidence, some studies have found correlations between having older siblings, who presumably bring in microbes, and being less likely to have allergies. Similarly, owning a pet dog (but not a cat) has been correlated with less eczema and, presumably, less allergy risk. That said, other studies of kids growing up on farms reportedly suggest exposure to animals does not affect prevalence of food allergies. (Farm kids do seem to have a lower incidence of asthma and hay fever, however.)

Lack of sunlight and lack of exposure to pathogens and/or symbiotic microbes are considered top theories for the rise in so-called modern diseases. These include food and environmental allergies, asthma, autoimmune disorders, and some types of cancer. Happily, both theories point in one direction, and it is the direction I most often give to my kids: *Go outside and play!*

Diet: Ancestrally, Prenatally, and in Infancy

When I was pregnant with Clara, not only did I eat eggs for lunch three times a week, my husband and I concocted a dinner party made entirely of egg dishes. And while the dinner party never came to fruition, plenty of the dish tasting did: pisco sours topped with egg-white froth, savory soufflés, salmon and asparagus with hollandaise, individual meringue pies. I abstained from the pisco sours but was otherwise quite drawn to any egg dish I could find. And nuts—especially cashews and almonds, the ones Clara was later deemed particularly allergic to—were my favorite snack. Did my indulgences cause Clara's allergies?

Fifteen years ago, I would have been told yes. Back then, women were advised in a blanket manner to avoid allergens while pregnant and breast-feeding. However, no evidence has since emerged to support the claim that maternal avoidance helps. Quite the contrary. Some researchers suggest this advice may have even helped increase food allergy rates. There are currently no mainstream recommendations for pregnant women to avoid eating major allergens.

That doesn't mean mothers are off the hook. A review of forty-two studies found a link between eating significant quantities of hydrogenated oils (i.e., trans fats), such as those found in fast food, while pregnant and an increased risk of allergic disease. And diets high in fresh produce, olive oil, fish, yogurt, legumes, and whole grains may have a protective effect against allergies.

And, of course, smoking is bad. Smoking during pregnancy and exposure to secondhand smoke has been correlated with higher allergy rates. Cigarettes or possibly other environmental toxins could have an epigenetic effect on genes that is passed on through at least two generations, according to a 2014 review article in the journal *Allergy, Asthma and Clinical Immunology*. That is, the smoking habit of a grandparent or great-grandparent could make a child more likely to develop asthma or allergies— even if the two have never met.

What the baby eats is likely most critical. Breast-feeding for at least six months or up to a year has also been correlated with fewer allergies and less risk of asthma, although if it cuts down the range of foods the older baby eats, especially allergens, it might be counterproductive.

Over a decade ago, some studies suggested that avoiding certain foods in infancy would help decrease the risk of allergies but follow-up studies failed to find a protective effect. The first studies may have been "contaminated by confounding," write scientists Katrina J. Allen and Jennifer J. Koplin in *Food Allergy: Adverse Reactions to Foods and Food Additives*, where another variable, beyond avoidance, likely explains the erroneous association.

Reversing these early studies, avoiding allergens has now been correlated with actually increasing the prevalence of food allergies. Here are just a few examples: Delaying the introduction of eggs until age 1 was linked to a five-fold increase of egg allergy, according to a study by Koplin and Allen published in the *Journal of Allergy and Clinical Immunology*. Similarly, delaying the introduction of cereal grain until after six months of age has been associated with increased risk of grain allergies. And providing support in the converse, regular fish consumption before age one has been associated with decreased risk of fish allergies.

Avoiding allergens in infancy may increase the risk of food allergy development.

The take-home message from these and a wide range of further studies being published in various countries across the globe is simple: Most of us should be feeding our kids allergens early, carefully, and often.

Skin and Gut Disconnect

Arguably one of the more compelling theories, proposed by Dr. Lack in 1998, is currently the dual-exposure hypothesis, which posits that food allergies arise when an infant's skin is exposed to allergens, via household dust or on a caregiver's hands, but the mouth and gut are not. The skin and gut then send contradictory information to the immune system. The skin says, *Yes, I know it—and hate it*, while the mouth and gut say, *Never heard of it.* This disconnect, in some cases, causes a toddler's immune system to "decide" that the substance is not *meant* to be eaten. This makes sense, if you consider it from an evolutionary perspective. In many hunter-gatherer communities today, and thus what evolutionary biologists expect was the standard practice of our distant ancestors, any and all foods are, well, *eaten* and offered to babies to eat, albeit often in an already-been-chewed form. Over our evolutionary history, if a baby was coming in contact with a substance but was never offered it to eat, chances were it wasn't a food. Perhaps it was even poisonous.

How does an infant become exposed to allergens on their skin? Foods that are eaten in the baby's household, day care, or playgroup are found in trace amounts on the hands of parents and other caregivers, on tabletops, and even in household dust. Some studies testing this theory have looked at the allergen-protein content in the dust in babies' beds. Babies with eczema are particularly vulnerable to these exposures, as their skin is more permeable.

Doctors used to think eczema was *caused* by food allergies, but they are now beginning to understand that it may be more complicated than that. Eczema appears to be promoting the development of allergies and possibly asthma as well.

In many cases, eczema is caused by a dysfunctional or mutated gene that is supposed to encode profilaggrin, a protein responsible for making the outer layer of skin healthy. More specifically, profilaggrin affects the skin's pH, moisture level, and possibly even antimicrobial activity. If her body does not produce enough profilaggrin, an infant suffers what scientists call "epithelial barrier dysfunction." Food proteins can more easily cross the damaged skin and find their way, with the help of butlerlike, androgen-presenting cells, to the immune system's T or B cells. These cells correctly say, "Hey, food protein, you are not supposed to be here!" This triggers an immune response, including production of IgE, in an effort to get the allergen out. Interestingly, this reaction is believed to have originally evolved as a mechanism to fight invasive parasites.

In an at-risk toddler, an allergen can be like the new kid at school waiting for approval from the popular and powerful immune system. The immune system asks the opinions of the skin and the gut: Is the peanut friend or foe? The gut is predisposed, of course, to like food. And the gut tends to have more sway—unless, of course, it has never met the allergen and holds no opinion whatsoever. In that case, the soft-voiced, food-phobic skin has the upper hand and the immune system sides against the allergen.

But if the gut has some experience with the protein, due to early and regular introduction in infancy, the immune system pacifies the skin's erroneous warning signals with regulatory immune responses that turn off IgE production. The food is labeled "friend" and, with continued gut exposure, no allergy develops.

If, however, there continues to be no gut education about specific proteins (i.e., the baby is not allowed to eat substances that she is coming across on her skin) over enough months, the immune system is left listening only to the skin's mistrust of the food allergen, perhaps even to the point of paranoia. When it first sees this mysterious compound coming through the front gate (mouth), it may launch a full-scale attack.

Studies supporting this theory include those done in mice and humans. In mice, placing egg white or peanut proteins onto damaged skin led to allergy-type immune responses. In humans, food allergen–specific T cells have been found on the skin of people with eczema. A large study that followed infants from birth to childhood found that those whose inflamed skin was treated with peanut oil as babies were more likely to be allergic to peanuts by the age of five. I look at the almond oil ingredient in my favorite hand lotion and wonder, did this contribute to Clara's severe almond allergy?

The dual-exposure hypothesis also explains a lot of the geographical differences found among the prevalence rates of different food allergies. Where certain foods are rarely found within a home, and thus no dust, table smears, or sticky fingers could be created for infant skin contact, allergies to that food are also rare. But if the food is popular in the home and culture, but the baby isn't given it to eat, allergies arise. For example, in Singapore, there is a common allergy to bird's nest soup and in Hong Kong, royal jelly allergy is prevalent. Kiwi allergy was not an issue in the United Kingdom until it was introduced in the 1970s and 1980s, and now it is a top worry among allergists.

Similarly, this hypothesis predicts that in countries where a certain allergen is a prevalent and popular food *and* it is regularly given to babies to eat from a very early age, there would be low allergy rates to that food. And vice versa. In countries where an allergen is a popular food source, but babies are kept from eating it, we'd expect to see allergy rates rise.

And this is just what we see. In countries in Africa and Asia, where peanuts are eaten by everyone, including babies (obviously in a chewed or otherwise processed form), peanut allergy is rare. But in the United Kingdom, the United States, Canada, and Australia, where recommendations have encouraged delaying the introduction of peanuts until toddlerhood, peanut allergy rates have skyrocketed.

Geography can also affect the severity of allergy, possibly determined by the different ways an allergen is processed in the area. In the United States, peanut allergy sufferers react to different substances within a peanut than peanut allergy sufferers in Spain and Sweden do. One could try to argue there is a genetic difference to the reaction, but other studies, including the study of ten thousand Jewish children growing up in different locales detailed in the next section, suggest it has more to do with environment than ancestry.

That is not to say that genes don't play a strong role in the development of allergies. They do. Absolutely. Parents who have eczema or allergies of their own have babies who are at high risk for food allergies.

(Interestingly, it seems that another risk factor for eczema, and possibly food allergies as well, is having well-educated parents. It may not simply be that educated parents are more likely to get a diagnosis. Something more complicated is likely at work, although scientists aren't sure yet what it is. I can't help but think of the culturally prevalent stereotype of the wheezing, allergic brainiac. I always thought, well, the asthma and hay fever makes it hard for them to play sports so they read a lot instead. But perhaps I have it backward. When Harsha noted that Deelan exhibited shocking precocity on the piano as a toddler, and at school he is at the top of his class, I was not surprised.)

But not all high-risk babies go on to have problems. The genes open the door, possibly via eczema, but only certain environments push the kids through that door, perhaps by not protecting them through adequate exposures in the first place. The other theories could also play supportive roles. A sunlight-deprived, infectious-exposure-deprived, microbe-deprived immune system—that is, one maturing in the developed world—may be particularly vulnerable to the dual-allergen exposure tug-of-war.

Across the school courtyard from Harsha, with a son in Deelan's class, a daughter in Clara's class, and an eight-year-old boy in a different school, stands Zoe. Zoe is a wisp of an Englishwoman with short hair, a big heart, and often a worried expression on her pixie face. Her kids seem to get the worst of the illnesses that pass through the school, and I just assumed that they must have allergies as well. "No, nothing," she said. "Me, on the other hand, I am allergic to everything."

A few weeks prior to our conversation, Zoe had to call the paramedics in the middle of the night; an allergen hiding in a mixed juice drink was sending her into anaphylactic shock. Once, she had a reaction on an airplane and swelled so much in the face that she "looked like [she] had done a few rounds with Mike Tyson." Upon disembarkation, Ben, the kids' father, got taken in for questioning!

Ben is also an allergy sufferer. In addition to dealing with eczema, he carries an EpiPen with him everywhere due to a very severe Brazil nut allergy. But their kids are allergy-free.

When I expressed surprise, she explained that she had disregarded the UK government's advice when she was pregnant and when her kids were babies. Her sister, a nutrition researcher in Glasgow and fellow allergy sufferer, had advised her to embrace allergens rather than avoid them. (Zoe's sister's three children are allergy-free, too.) This advice made more sense to Zoe than the government's recommendations to restrict the types of food offered to infants and pregnant women, she said. With an understanding that was truly ahead of its time, Zoe explained that she wanted to expose her babies to allergens so that their bodies would know they were safe foods.

Particularly fearful of life-threatening nut allergies, due to her husband's condition, Zoe, who hates nuts, "ate them under duress," during all three pregnancies. She then breast-fed exclusively for six months, accepting this one recommendation from the United Kingdom's National Health Service, but tried to keep her diet varied. When each child was between six and seven months old, she introduced all major allergens including eggs, milk, whole wheat toast, and nuts. When her eldest, Raphael, broke out in a bright red rash after eating scrambled eggs, she continued giving him eggs in baked goods until the allergy disappeared when he was about two years old.

It is these early feeding experiences that Zoe credits with her kids' allergy-free bodies and lives. Considering the eczema each child suffered in infancy, this conjecture is likely accurate. "It just made sense to me that that is what the body would need," she said, talking about early exposure.

Today there is considerable research to back up her intuition.

IN AN ALLERGY-FREE NUTSHELL

1. The prevalence of severe food allergies is on a startling rise, doubling within the last decade.

   - Simultaneously, the number of hospitalizations for allergic reactions has increased sevenfold.

   - Nearly one in ten preschool children in developed countries, and 6 to 8 percent of all children worldwide, have a clinically documented food allergy.

2. The top theories for explaining this rise include:

   - Lack of exposure to sunshine, due to indoor lifestyles and possible overuse of sunblock.

   - Lack of exposure to pathogens and friendly microbes due to necessary sanitation processes in the developed world.

   - Delayed introduction of food allergens due to outdated recommendations.

Chapter 2

The Solution

Clues to the Cure

Dr. Gideon Lack became convinced something was amiss in 2003 when he was giving a talk in Israel in a large lecture hall filled with pediatricians and allergists. He asked the doctors to raise their hands if they had had a patient with peanut allergy in the last year. In the United Kingdom, where Lack practices, nearly every hand would have gone up. But in this audience, "something like three hands shot up," he told Jerome Groopman of *The New Yorker*. This startled Lack and he decided to investigate.

In 2008, he conducted a large, observational study of ten thousand Jewish children, half of whom were living in the United Kingdom and the other half in an ethnically and economically similar section of Israel. He and his fellow researchers found the rate of peanut allergy among the UK children was more than ten times that of those in Israel. Other allergies were also more prevalent among children in the London area: tree nut allergy was fourteen times more prevalent, sesame five times more, milk and egg two to three times more.

The study was designed to roughly control for genetics, leaving the environment to be the main difference between the two cohorts. Was there something causing the allergies in the United Kingdom or something protective in Israel?

The answer lay in a popular Israeli snack food called Bamba.

Parents from both countries in the study were surveyed and the researchers quickly learned that the main difference between the two cohorts was the timing in which peanuts were introduced. In Israel, infants had consumed peanut protein, usually via the peanut butter and puffed corn snack Bamba, before they were six months of age, whereas in England peanut products were not usually introduced until after the age of one.

According to Lack, there is a joke in Israel that the first three words a child learns are *abba* (father), *ima* (mother), and Bamba.

As noted in the previous chapter, countries in Asia and Africa that are known to have a low prevalence of peanut allergy also introduce peanuts into the diet quite early, often in the already-been-chewed form, spat from the mouth of the mother into the mouth of her child. (Saliva, a rich source of enzymes and antibodies, may offer some benefits to the infant.)

But in developed countries, quite the opposite had been taking place. In fact, governments and medical associations were specifically advising avoidance. For example, in 2000, following suit on the 1998 guidelines put forth by the United Kingdom's Department of Health, the American Academy of Pediatrics (AAP) mandated that children should wait until age one to try cow's milk and age two to taste eggs, and that they should not consume peanuts, shellfish, tree nuts, or fish until they had reached three years of age. Eight years later, the AAP backed away from these rules, saying there was little evidence that avoiding these foods prevented the development of food allergies. But they didn't give any new recommendations, leaving parents in the lurch, with many deciding to stick with the old guidelines, thinking they were playing it safe.

By 2013, there had been enough studies suggesting avoidance was helping cause the rise in allergies that the American Academy of Allergy, Asthma and Immunology (AAAAI) issued guidelines encouraging parents, via pediatricians, to introduce possible allergens to infants between four and six months old. Much of the medical community ignored these controversial recommendations, claiming the evidence was purely observational, even anecdotal. There needed to be proof via large intervention studies to be sure that early exposure was truly the best advice.

The first of such studies, Learning Early About Peanut (LEAP), came out in February 2015 with resounding results. More than five hundred infants, considered at high risk for peanut allergy, either due to severe eczema, egg allergy, or both, but not yet exhibiting peanut allergy as verified by clinical testing, were randomly divided into two groups. One group avoided peanut proteins and the other consumed at least 6 grams of peanut protein (the equivalent of about twenty-four peanuts offered via Bamba or peanut butter) every week over the course of three or more meals. The study, conducted by Dr. Lack's research team, started when the babies were between four and eleven months old. When they turned five years old, they were tested for food allergies. Early introduction of peanut among high-risk babies halted development of the allergy by 70 to 80 percent! A follow-up study, LEAP-On, showed that this tolerance continued even after the kids stopped eating peanuts regularly.

In a concurrent editorial in the *New England Journal of Medicine*, where the peanut study was published, new guidelines concerning peanuts were immediately called for and interim advice was offered for parents via pediatricians and allergists on the amount of peanut to introduce based on the child's age and risk of allergy. Dr. Lack, for his part, thinks babies, *especially* high-risk babies, should be regularly given peanut butter, assuming they are healthy and developmentally ready to eat solid foods, as early as three months of age—almost as if it were a vaccination against the allergy—but starting them on peanut butter after three months could be risky.

The second of such studies, Enquiring About Tolerance (EAT), was published in March 2016. While it followed a methodology

similar to the peanut study, it had twice the number of participants (1,303) and investigated six major allergens—cow's milk,
peanut, sesame, fish, wheat, and egg. And instead of looking just
at high-risk children, babies were selected from the general population. Importantly, babies were screened via clinical testing
to check whether they had *already* developed food allergies; if
they had, they were asked to avoid the allergen that was already
a problem but follow the recommendations for the other foods.

The thirteen hundred healthy, breast-fed three-month-old infants were randomly divided into two groups. One group, the
"standard introduction group," or the experiment's control, followed the United Kingdom's guidelines and delayed introducing
solids until after six months of age. The parents of the other half,
the "early introduction group," were asked to feed their babies allergens early, carefully, and often, and given specific guidelines
on how to do so.

Three years later, the now toddlers were tested for allergies.
The results were analyzed in two ways: intention to treat and
per protocol. The intention-to-treat analysis compared the two
groups and found that the early exposure group had slightly but
nonsignificantly less food allergies than the standard introduction group. The per-protocol analysis looked more carefully at
the early exposure group, dividing it further into two subgroups:
those that actually followed the recommendations to expose
early and often (that is, they followed the "protocol") and those
that didn't. The results of the protocol-following group were then
examined in detail.

The 208 kids who had been systematically exposed to food
allergens—early and often—were significantly less likely to develop a food allergy. Compared to the control group, they were
67 percent less likely to have any food allergy at three years old.

The effect was particularly strong for egg and peanut allergy.
Only 1.4 percent of adequately exposed kids developed an egg allergy, compared to 5.5 percent of the control group, and none de-

veloped a peanut allergy, compared to 2.5 percent of the control. Moreover, there was a dose response relationship between the amount of egg and peanut eaten and the risk of developing an allergy. The more eggs and peanut butter a baby ate, the less likely she was to develop an egg or peanut allergy by toddlerhood.

There was not a single case of anaphylactic shock in the study, proving that it is safe to introduce potential allergens to three-month-old babies. This is an important finding, showing that most parents have been needlessly avoiding these foods in infancy, said Dr. James Baker, the chief medical officer of FARE, who was not involved in the study. A reaction is unlikely at this early age, and if one does occur, it is most likely to be minor. That said, if your baby has dry skin, eczema, or is otherwise considered high risk, it is best to have her evaluated by an allergist before introducing potential allergens at home. The study also found that early exposure to solids did not alter breast-feeding duration.

The lack of adherence to the early exposure recommendations was an unexpected finding. Despite regular follow-up appointments, calls from the study's dietician, and a requirement to keep a weekly food log, fewer than half of the parents who were asked to expose their baby to allergens early and often actually did so.

Why? Could it be that the parents who didn't follow the guidelines did so because their kids were actually already allergic? The researchers wondered this, too, and tested these kids at three years old to find out if they had greater than average prevalence of food allergy. They didn't. Nor was there a link between kids at high risk to developing a food allergy and adherence to the guidelines.

There was a link, however, between *parent-perceived* allergy and failure to follow the guidelines. This is an important point. Parents are so scared of severe allergic attacks that the slightest suggestion of a reaction (e.g., "Mason became fussy after eating

Dose-Response Analysis of the Relationship Between Weekly Dose Consumed and Resulting Allergy

These graphs plot the prevalence of peanut allergy and egg allergy (panel A), or sensitization to peanut and egg, as found by skin-prick testing, at twelve months (panel B) and thirty-six months (panel C), against the mean weekly consumption of peanut and egg protein in the first six months of life. The prevalence of both food allergy and positive skin-prick tests diminish with increasing levels of weekly consumption. In other words, the more exposure a baby had, the less likely she was to have problems with that food in toddlerhood. Insets show the same data on an enlarged y axis.

Reprinted with permission from Michael R. Perkin, Kirsty Logan, Anna Tseng, Bunmi Raji, Salma Ayis, Janet Peacock, Helen Brough, et al., "Randomized Trial of Introduction of Allergenic Foods in Breast-Fed Infants," *New England Journal of Medicine* 374 (2016): 1733–43, doi:10.1056/NEJMoa1514210.

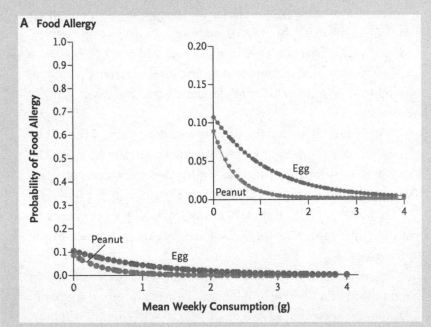

A   Food Allergy

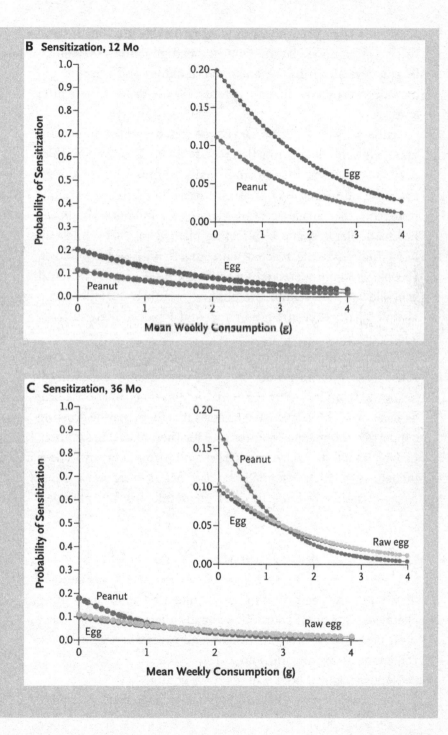

scrambled eggs") causes them to restrict their kids' diets. This fear is compounded by the now outdated guidelines to keep allergens away from babies and small children and continues to play a powerful role in how parents choose to feed their little ones.

While we were talking, Dr. Baker raised another important point. He said his organization, Food Allergy Research and Education (FARE), had heard from many parents who misunderstood the LEAP and EAT studies. Not realizing that the studies tested and then made accommodations for infants who *already* had food allergies, and also feeling blamed for their child's allergy, many parents reacted with anger. But, said Dr. Baker, "People should understand that it is not their fault. . . . Even if you follow [the prevention protocol], your child could still end up allergic." Early exposure is a helmet and a padded body suit, not a force field.

Within six months from the LEAP study's publication, a consensus on "interim guidelines" concerning early exposure to peanut were endorsed by the AAP and ten other major medical associations. This consensus suggests that there may be growing support in the medical community for the broader recommendations issued by AAAAI concerning all major allergens. These guidelines—which essentially say *feed babies allergens early and often*—may save millions of kids from developing food allergies.

But She's Already Allergic

So we are now beginning to know quite a bit about preventing allergies, but what if your kid is already allergic? Have all these great new advances in our understanding of allergy onset just come too late for you and your kid?

No. Especially if he is still relatively young.

The newest treatment, which is being pioneered by experts

at Northwestern University in Chicago, involves educating the immune system on the safety of, say, peanuts, by attaching peanut proteins to white blood cells. This interaction safely helps the immune system learn to accept peanuts in the same way we might cordially befriend the friend of our best friend. So far, the research has only been done in mice, but the researchers are hopeful the technique will transfer to humans.

Already at work in humans are the various versions of oral immunotherapy, briefly discussed in the previous chapter, where the immune system is reeducated through the mouth and gut by asking the patient to eat the offending substance in small graduated amounts. When I made a cake for Clara with just one egg and gave her one-twentieth every day, I was performing oral immunotherapy.

For the small minority of allergy sufferers who have extremely severe intolerance to certain foods—those who react to the tiniest trace amounts, such as contaminants from factory machinery or who go into anaphylactic shock simply from touching an allergen—Dr. Kari Nadeau of Stanford University has successfully developed an oral immunotherapy treatment that is basically a slower, even more careful version of what we did for Clara.

Nadeau had medical-grade flours made of common allergens so that they can be eaten in *extremely* tiny amounts on a daily basis. The amount is upped slowly, sometimes backtracking a bit when the kid reacts, but barreling ahead no matter, until the formerly allergic child can safely tolerate a full dose of the allergen, say a small handful of nuts or an entire egg. They must continue eating this "maintenance dose" every day, for possibly the rest of their lives.

In the vast majority of situations, the child, especially if young and allergic to dairy or egg, does not need commercial-grade powders but can start with the actual allergen in its food form in minute amounts, slowly introducing greater and greater quantities until it is no longer an issue. They then need to eat a maintenance dose of the formerly offending food two to three times a week for at least five years. My kids, like most allergic children, fall into this camp.

At this time, allergy desensitization, to be done safely, requires intense hands-on help from a doctor. Do not "go it alone" if your child has major food allergies. Approach a doctor as soon as possible about desensitization through oral immunotherapy, especially if the child is allergic to dairy or egg. The younger your child, the more likely the treatment will work.

Unfortunately, desensitization protocols for nuts, seeds, fish, and shellfish are still in their infancy and are likely unavailable in most medical practices. It may be helpful, however, to stop avoiding all nuts if your child is only allergic to, say, almonds. Or all fish if only halibut is a problem. Have a new round of specific testing done first, to find out if any new allergies have developed. Any allergenic foods deemed safe for your child should be given to her regularly. You might also want to ride the current wave of ongoing research in allergy desensitization. Information on how to participate in a clinical trial is available in the resource section at the back of this book.

When approaching a doctor, keep in mind that he may not be used to being taught something by his patients. And in harried practices, the change in the usual dynamic could be mistaken as confrontation. It can be useful to acknowledge how new this information is. Bring with you a copy of this book or download and print out some of the studies mentioned here, which are linked from this book's page on my website (RobinNixonPompa.com). Be deferential, open minded, and firm: "If I were a doctor, I'd hate it when people self-prescribe remedies, but this approach seems to be getting a lot of attention in the media and I can't help but wonder if it might help my child."

If you get resistance, listen carefully to the reasons. Are they about your specific child? Perhaps your child has compounding issues or has passed outside the critical age window? Or does it sound as if your doctor simply feels uncomfortable or uninformed about the new research?

If there are concerns about your child's suitability, thank your doctor and consider getting a second opinion. If the concerns seem more about the doctor, perhaps try from a different angle: "I'd really like to learn more about this approach and find a safe way to try it with my child. Is this something you have the time to help me with? If not, do you know someone who might be interested?" You then have a platform to partner with a medical professional, learn together about the latest science, and hopefully resolve your child's allergies.

Making the Medicine Go Down

In either case—whether you are working with a doctor to desensitize a child or to prevent allergies from developing—compliance is the major impediment. At-risk and allergic kids often associate allergens with feeling sick, or at least an unpleasant taste, and they are naturally repulsed by the idea of eating it. (I can relate; I won't even walk into the restaurant that gave me food poisoning a couple years ago, let alone eat there.) The older children in Nadeau's studies often come up with clever ways to try to disguise the taste. Mixing the flours with ice cream is popular.

With younger children, parents may need to be even more creative. When my son Arthur was a small infant, he would break out in hives whenever anyone kissed him after eating eggs themselves. When I consulted with Dr. Lack, a kind and composed Englishman, he became uncharacteristically agitated when he heard the infrequency of my attempts to feed Arthur egg. "Egg allergy needs to be treated seriously!" he said, slapping the back of his hand, which I took as his gentlemanly substitute for pounding the table.

Poor Arthur. Following Dr. Lack's advice, the hives quickly

subsided, but Arthur, usually an amiable baby with an admirable appetite, would cry and swat my spoon away, sending puree all over the counter and floor whenever I tried to feed him egg. These experiences led to the discovery of many of the tricks and recipes detailed in this book that helped both of us persevere.

And let me admit, it can be hard to persevere, day after day, week after week. I don't *want* to force food down my kids' throats. Let's have a peaceful house, and especially a peaceful table, I find myself silently pleading.

But I also don't want to start carrying an EpiPen again. As Melanie Thernstrom wrote in a *New York Times* article, "Food allergies amplify a kind of fear every parent experiences—of a child dashing suddenly into the street and, just like that, being gone. Your child is always playing near a precipice that is visible only to you: you may be able to keep her from falling off, but you can never move her away from the edge."

This stress alone is enough to motivate me most of the time. Imagining my kids in college enjoying a well-earned restaurant brunch without a care in the world is another powerful motivator. And if I am really struggling with fatigue, I extrapolate from the most cutting-edge research and imagine that treating my kids' allergies will perhaps—through an epigenetic twist—keep my grandkids and great-grandkids from getting sick as well. With this encouraging thought, I stay up, make the nut butter, and prep yet another batch of "hidden-egg pancakes," feeling hopeful that my family will stay allergy-free for generations to come.

IN AN ALLERGY-FREE NUTSHELL

1. Babies who are exposed to food allergens *early and often* may be protected from food allergies.

2. Why "early"? For most babies, exposing them to allergens when they are between three and six months old is safe, as few have yet had time to develop food allergies. Check with a doctor first if the baby has dry skin, eczema, or a family history of allergies.

3. Why "often"? It is believed that if the immune system is not regularly exposed to potential food allergens, a food allergy could develop.

4. Already allergic? Approach a doctor about exploring allergy desensitization through graduated amounts, especially in the cases of egg and dairy allergy.

5. The younger the child, the better the chance of finding relief from food allergies.

6. For everyone's benefit, find ways to make allergens palatable.

7. If your child ends up food allergic, don't blame yourself. Sometimes there is nothing that can be done.

Chapter 3

Implementing at Home

While scientists are still debating the various causes of the dramatic rise in food allergies, parents may now be able to help curb it. Whether it is first-world sanitation, insufficient sunshine, or some other modern phenomenon at the root of the escalating problem, it ultimately doesn't matter for you and your family. What matters is finding a way to protect your little ones. And on that point, with the completion of several large, significant studies (see chapter 2), scientists and doctors are in many cases eating their previous recommendations and slowly starting to agree on the best methods to prevent food allergies.

We can likely curb the rise in food allergies simply by feeding our kids allergens early and often.

In the following sections, I will outline exactly how to do that at different stages in your child's development. But please, particularly for at-risk infants—those with dry skin, eczema, or a family history of allergies—speak with an allergist before introducing allergens. Tests may show that it would be safest to introduce certain foods in a hospital. But once your child has been given the all clear—with the caveat that they eat allergens two or three times a week—turn to this book with abandon.

This book is not meant to be a sole resource in feeding practices. While much of the information goes beyond allergy prevention, its primary focus is on food allergies, so you may want to turn to other sources for general nutritional advice—especially if you feel worried about your own food habits and nutrition.

Lastly, please don't let anything in this book give succor to the guilt and stress monsters that plague all parents. The aim of this book is to make things easier, not harder!

Pregnancy Through the Newborn Stage

An unborn infant is basically sterile. I know, how can I use the word *sterile* for the adorable pudge of rapidly growing baby we see on ultrasound scans, but it is true. He is as clean as he will ever be while he is still inside his mother's body. And I am not just talking about the dirt and crumbs that seem to attack my children within minutes of leaving the bathtub. A newborn, before he takes leave of his mother, is free of all bacteria. As he emerges, he is quickly colonized by nearby microbes, usually those of the mother, especially when the birth is vaginal. As he is pushed through the birth canal, a newborn gathers beneficial bacteria that babies born by C-section miss out on. Scientists are now realizing that this early bacterial colonization is so important that some are studying whether C-section babies could be helped by simply being immediately wiped with birth canal bacteria gathered from the mother with a bit of gauze.

Most doctors, allergists included, recommend breast-feeding in early infancy.

For no one really wants to stay as "clean" as we are in our mother's womb. We need our microbes; they are our "old friends" (see chapter 1). We have lived in secret symbiosis with them for thousands of years, nourishing and supporting one another.

By the time a new mother and father are peering for the first time into the face of the little being they have created, the infant has already met and befriended millions of microbes. These tiny organisms "set up shop" on the baby's skin and digestive system and become the nascent immune system's first teachers. From here on, anything the baby comes in contact with—via skin, mouth, or even eyes—will teach the infant immune system about the outside world.

So how do we make sure this education gets off on the right track? The most correct answer is: Nobody knows.

As a society, we tend to put a lot of weight on firsts. Early experiences are blamed or credited for a disproportionately large amount of later experiences. I've taken to asking parents if their kids have allergies, and if I am told no, I ask, "Why not?" This is usually met with laughter—and then I get a theory: "Oh, I ate really well while pregnant," or "I hardly breast-fed," or "I nursed him till he was two."

The research on breast-feeding is mixed, with some studies concluding that breast milk protects a kid from allergy development and other studies actually finding an association between nursing and food allergies, especially when breast-feeding is prolonged.

Do not needlessly avoid allergens while pregnant or lactating.

But food allergies are only one part of your child's overall health. And breast-feeding has been associated with so many positives—from protecting babies from infections, obesity, and diabetes to possibly increasing their IQ and later earning potential—*that most doctors, allergists included, recommend breast-feeding at this stage.* If you cannot breast-feed, or find it an overwhelming stressor, a high-quality formula can be substituted.

Regardless, at this stage, it is most important to respond to the baby's cues. He will tell you when he wants to eat and how much. Some babies are fast, some slow. Some like to suck, even after full. This is a time of learning about your baby. And a time for your baby to learn that he is safe. There is warmth and food available to his small vulnerable body. He will be protected.

The first twelve weeks of a baby's life are often called the fourth trimester, the theory being that human newborns, when compared to other species, are born developmentally premature. If women did not need to walk upright, our bodies would be shaped differently, in a way that could accommodate a larger infant. Instead, the baby comes out early and is in need of near constant comforting and sustenance during the newborn stage.

If you are pregnant or breast-feeding, do not avoid allergens, unless, of course, you are allergic to them. It is not clear whether how mothers eat while pregnant and breast-feeding directly affects allergy development or not. But it is clear that recommendations to avoid peanuts, tree nuts, eggs, soy, dairy, wheat, or other possible allergens, such as kiwi, during pregnancy and breast-feeding are pointless. And perhaps even harmful. So eat up!

Three to Five Months of Age: The Golden Window

Your baby is exiting the fourth trimester and is now, in the words of one mother I spoke with, "a proper baby." There is a bit of baby fat, and best of all, there are smiles. The baby shows an increased interest in the world. Perhaps her immune system does, too.

Many organizations, including UNICEF and the World Health Organization, recommend waiting to introduce solid foods (i.e., pureed foods) until the baby is six months old. In third-world countries, breast-feeding exclusively protects a vulnerable infant from possibly contaminated food and water. In the first world, early weaning has been associated with obesity.

....

Early exposure to allergens likely protects a baby from developing allergies in toddlerhood.

....

But if your aim is to avoid food allergies, this is the time period when many allergists are now saying to pounce, at the very least for peanut. The evidence is now suggesting this may be the golden window for introducing other major allergens as well.

Again, if allergies run in your baby's family history, or if he has eczema or dry skin, first have him evaluated by an allergist. Most likely, the doctor will want to give your baby a skin-prick test. This sounds more irritating than it is. It involves a nurse holding a baby's arm still (this is the part they usually hate most) while they write on it with a normal pen: *peanut, egg, milk, latex,* and so on. Then a tiny drop of the corresponding allergen is placed next to its written label. The drop is then pierced with a pin that enables a minuscule amount of the allergen to enter the skin.

I've tried it. If you are imagining the pain from a sewing needle slipping as you mend a button, stop. It is much duller than that, more akin to the "prick" of a stiff tag in a shirt. My babies, two of whom seemed particularly sensitive and reactive to the slightest irritation, have never minded the pricks. Clara even found the process fascinating: "Look at the little bubbles on my arm!" As a toddler, she liked to play nurse by happily drawing on her dolls' arms. My two boys were just annoyed at being held still.

After the pricks are done, you will be asked to wait five to twenty minutes. At least one round red circle will appear on your baby's arm. This is the control. If it doesn't react, the test has been done improperly. Large red circles around the other sites may indicate a developing food allergy. The nurse or doctor will inspect and measure these circles and give you advice from there.

Let's Say the Allergist Gives You the All Clear—Time to Start Feeding!

A main source of nutrition will continue to be breast milk or formula, but start introducing allergens immediately. You may want to start with other conventional baby's first foods, such as pureed oats, rice, vegetables, and fruits. This will help you evaluate your baby's swallowing technique and judge her readiness for solids. In particular, babies born prematurely may not be ready for solids at this stage.

As soon as possible, move on to the major allergens: eggs, wheat, cow's milk, peanuts, sesame, and fish. (See chapter 4 for specific guidance for each allergen.) Try to have them all introduced before five months of age. The earlier, the better.

To introduce a new food, try mixing it with breast milk or formula.

You may also want to introduce shellfish, tree nuts, and kiwi. It is expected that the principle of educating the immune system early and often with common allergens will hold for these allergens as well. However, they have not, at this time, been properly tested. It is possible that one may be an outlier and that early introduction will not protect the child from developing an allergy to that food down the line. Nevertheless, for most babies, it is perfectly safe to introduce these foods in early infancy, and there is a large chance that doing so will turn out to be protective.

Introduce one allergen at a time, paying attention to any signs of allergy. Food allergies are rare, but not unheard of, before five months old. In the unlikely case there is a reaction, it is equally unlikely to be dangerous at this age. Keep an eye out for hives, rashes, or wheezing that appear immediately after eating or coming in contact with a particular food. If your baby does have a reaction, consult with an allergist.

At this stage, your baby cannot chew and so everything must be pureed very well, with plenty of liquid, until the mixture is of a very smooth and runny consistency. Thinning a puree with breast milk or formula is a good way to make it more palatable to an infant. Mixing allergens with other popular foods, such as pureed steamed carrots or squash, can also be a good idea.

If your baby is fine with cow's milk, mixing an allergen with plain yogurt helps protect them from two allergies at once (dairy and the added allergen). All three of my kids loved plain yogurt at this stage and would eat really anything (especially spinach, go figure) if it was mixed with yogurt. I'd recommend avoiding thick Greek yogurt in the earliest months as it can be harder to swallow than the runnier stuff.

....

Pretending to eat some puree yourself will catch your baby's attention.

....

Use a flat spoon, one in which the indentation is very shallow, preferably of a material like wood or bisphenol A (BPA)–free plastic, which will give a little if the baby chomps down on it. You can also use your own (clean) fingers, letting a baby suck puree off them or even smearing a bit on their gums. Eating a bit yourself, or pretending to, can do wonders in catching an infant's interest in a new food.

After introducing each allergen, try to work up to the weekly doses provided below, preferably spaced over at least two days. These doses may be tweaked as research advances, but for now these are the best estimates we have. For additional dairy, sesame, and wheat options, please see chapter 4.

Weekly Guidelines for Preventing Food Allergies

- 2 1.5-ounce (40 g) containers plain yogurt or dairy equivalent (full fat for children under two years old)

- 1 small egg

- 3 rounded teaspoons peanut butter (use smooth, not chunky, for babies) or 5 teaspoons ground peanuts

- 3 teaspoons tahini or sesame equivalent

- 0.9 ounce (25 g) fish (about ¼ of an adult serving)

- 1 slice whole wheat bread or wheat equivalent

Work up to these amounts as fast or as slow as your baby wants. Some babies take to real food immediately, whereas others prefer breast milk or formula. It may be easier to divide the weekly amounts by seven and give them daily. This approach can help in keeping track of what has been given and is also beneficial at the earliest stages when the infant's daily capacity for real food is very small.

Allow your baby to set the pace.

If you are having trouble generating your baby's appetite for real food, try to offer food a little before you would normally nurse them. If you wait until they are very hungry, they may be too upset to actually eat. But if you can get some food into them before they even realize they are hungry, they will eat out of curiosity. And then you can nurse them at their normal time. You don't want to offer allergens after nursing or a bottle, as the baby will be full—or asleep!

Please don't worry that exposing your baby to solids at this stage will drastically reduce the amount of breast milk your baby drinks or that you may be accelerating weaning beyond your comfort level. It is true that the baby will no longer be *exclusively* breast-fed once other foods are introduced, but this term may be losing value, and in practice, it is rarely done for more than a few months; one large recent survey estimated that only 4 percent of babies are exclusively breast-fed at six months of age. Early exposure to allergenic foods in the EAT study was found to have no adverse effects on breast-feeding duration, with 97 percent of mothers in the early exposure group still breast-feeding when their baby was six months old, significantly exceeding national UK averages, where the study was conducted.

It can get cumbersome to keep track of the amounts, and babies are finicky and unpredictable. Three quarters of your carefully measured puree ends up in your baby's hair or in a crevice on his neck. Argh. Can you count it? Sadly no. This is a case where you did all the work and get none of the credit. The food does actually have to get in the baby. Don't lose heart. Even getting a little bit into the mouth is vastly better than none at all. So persevere and don't worry too much about the actual amounts at this stage. Just keep them in mind as a goal, hopefully to be achieved by the end of your baby's fifth month.

And unless you have one of those mythical babies that sleep through the night, you are probably not at your cognitive best. When Grant was this age, I left the house several times still in my slippers, and once in the middle of the night, I ordered cat food for a cat that existed purely in my imagination. I certainly couldn't remember if I gave the baby tahini on Monday.

Keep a weekly checklist until feeding the recommended amounts becomes routine.

It can really help to write it down. I know. You don't have time to write something down. But do it anyway, even if it is on a whiteboard in your kitchen, using the note function on your phone or a diet app, or by using the checklists provided in the back of this book.

Once all the allergens have been introduced, you can simplify your life by combining many of the allergens into a single puree and serving it at least twice a week. Tahini-yogurt-fish, anybody? Many of the recipes in this book do just this. My eggy pancakes protect kids from eggs and dairy at once. Make them with whole wheat flour and you get a leg up on wheat allergy as well. My salmon sliders, made with whole wheat bread crumbs and several eggs, battle three allergies at once as well. A list of such powerhouse recipes can be found on page 99.

If you are looking for the simplest way to protect your baby from food allergies, try the Kiwi EAT Wheaty Mix & Mash with mixed tree nut butter, a dish concocted by the EAT study researchers and tweaked by me. Eight major food allergies— egg, dairy, wheat, peanut, tree nut, fish, kiwi, and sesame—are addressed by this baby meal. Make this variation of the recipe, provided on page 201, and make sure your baby eats all of it over at least two days. Job done.

In addition to the puree recipes, which specifically target this age group, many of the proper food recipes in this book can be modified for the younger baby. Simply leave out any salt, sugar, or honey and puree until smooth. *(Note: Honey may contain bacteria that can't be handled by the digestive system of a child less than one year old, so recipes containing honey should not be served to babies.)* This technique can be particularly helpful if you have toddlers/preschoolers to feed as well as a baby, allowing you to make one meal for everyone. I often puree my older kids' leftovers to give to my infant the next day. With this in mind, salt can be added to individual plates, rather than in the cooking process or on the serving platter. This way, when the leftovers get pureed, they won't be too salty for baby.

Five to Nine Months

Okay. Now things get fun. Your baby is learning to sit, and if you thought she was cute before, oh boy, now she is really cute. And life is getting a wee bit easier. You may be more sleep deprived than ever, so it may not *feel* easier, but once your baby can sit and use her hands, things do, on the most practical level, get a bit easier. She will likely leave your side, for at least a few minutes, to play on the floor, freeing up your hands to, well, prepare her lunch.

> **While purees should be getting lumpier, keeping the allergen smooth may help it go down.**

By this age, hopefully the doses are now easily eaten each week. If you are having trouble meeting the recommended amounts, don't worry. Just continue to use the checklists and encourage your child to eat the food by repeated exposure or by trying different recipes to make a food more palatable. Also continue to keep an eye out for signs of allergy (hives, immediate vomiting, wheezing) and contact a pediatrician or allergist if you are worried.

At this age, the baby is hearing an internal drumbeat: Learn to use hands, learn to use hands. So if you place finger foods to play with in front of the baby's high chair, she will be excited about mealtime. Bits of cereal, diced fruits, and vegetables (avoiding skins and seeds), and small bits of soft toast with spread are great. I also like to cut long sticklike pieces of cucumbers, peppers, and carrots and keep them cold for a teething baby to gnaw on. Give them only when you will be sitting with the baby in the unlikely event she is able to break off a piece that she could choke on. And while we are talking about choking hazards, avoid or slice round foods, such as cherry tomatoes, grapes, and blue-berries, which can get lodged in an infant's throat. Never give a baby a whole nut.

Your baby will likely try to feed herself these finger foods, opening her mouth wide, and often failing to get any of the smaller pieces into her mouth. See the wide-open mouth as an allergy-prevention opportunity. Have your spoon at the ready and whisk it in.

(Please note: In general, it is best to respect your baby's cues rather than sneak in a spoonful of puree. I only recommend this approach if you are having trouble getting your baby to eat a particular allergen.)

Purees should be getting gradually lumpier at this stage, but if your baby hates one of the allergens, keeping that puree extra smooth may help in getting it down. If your baby wants your spoon, let her have it and get another one. She can experiment with feeding herself, and while she is distracted, you can pop in more allergen puree!

Expect a mess, of course. When you are most tired of cleaning, comfort yourself by repeating: This stage will not last forever. It really won't. Take pictures!

Make sure to offer your older baby different textures as well as different foods, slowly going from puree to a more mashed consistency. Babies adjust to these changes differently; again, allow your baby to set the pace.

It can be comforting (but by all means not essential) for both you and your baby to feed her puree before a family meal and then give her additional finger foods at the table when everyone is eating. This way, you know she is getting adequate nutrition and is being protected from allergy development *and* she is also being exposed to family foods. Plus, you can hold your own fork, rather than a baby spoon during the meal, and possibly have a chance to eat something yourself.

Nine to Twelve Months

Much of the above also pertains to this stage. Food should be getting lumpier and lumpier. Some babies have a tooth or two by now, but even if yours doesn't, his gums will be hard enough to do some of the mashing himself. Cutting soft foods into long sticklike shapes (the size of thick-cut fries) is particularly popular, allowing the older baby to feed himself to some degree.

Continue to offer small finger foods, too. He will be getting more successful at putting these into his mouth. He may particularly like textures that fall apart in his mouth, like hamburger and fish, potatoes, and hard-boiled eggs. As he works his tongue around these shapes, he is strengthening this muscle, which in turn will help him form different and more complex sounds. That's right, as he is learning to eat, he is also getting ready to learn to talk.

**Introduce all major allergens and
as many different foods as possible before
the baby can crawl.**

All the major allergens can be offered in these friendly shapes, in addition to purees. This is particularly important because babies, somewhere between seven and fifteen months, can suddenly become disdainful of purees or resent being spoon fed. Whole wheat toast, spread with a bit of peanut butter, Greek yogurt, or tahini, can be cut into bite-size squares or hand-size sticks. Omelets can be fried nearly crispy and cut small or long. Some babies this age like a medium-hard cheese, such as cheddar, sliced thin. Ripe kiwis or hard-boiled eggs, peeled and quartered lengthwise, may be enjoyed. Wheat cereals (look for Weetabix) can be particularly convenient since they travel well and need no preparation. *Here, sweetie, chew on this.* See the subsequent chapters for more allergen-specific ideas.

Many babies, at the later part of this period, become mobile. Whether it is by crawling (often backward at first) or a butt scoot or some precocious walking, little ones start to figure out how to get from point A to point B. This new mobility may be accompanied by a restriction in how willing he or she is to try new foods—and this may be a good thing.

The theory is, over our evolutionary history, babies who can't yet walk or crawl are unlikely to come across poisons. Anything near them is likely vetted by a caring adult and the baby safely puts just about everything in his mouth. But once he can get around by himself, he can get himself into trouble. He might happen upon a poisonous plant, a spider, or a potential choke hazard. So it is time for the instinct to put everything in his mouth to take a backseat.

This is one of the reasons it is a good idea to introduce as many foods as possible *before* this stage. Before babies are mobile, they are willing to try nearly anything. And if the food is already familiar at nine months, they are unlikely to reject it later (until mid-toddlerhood, that is; see the next section). Also, the immune system should be more willing to accept these new foods as safe at this early premobile stage. In addition to allergens, I have found it particularly valuable to introduce bitter vegetables, such as leafy greens, broccoli, and other members of the cabbage family, before a baby is mobile. Bitterness can be a sign of poison, so unless a baby is already familiar with the taste as a safe food, it can be hard to help him enjoy the taste as he gets older.

This theory also underscores the logic behind early exposure to allergens. The immune system is more wary, even paranoid, in the older baby and toddler. If this is when it first encounters, say, peanut butter, it may overreact. It may declare the food a poison and a full-scale allergic response could result.

If your child does show signs of a developing food allergy—

such as hives, a runny or blocked nose, itchy eyes, throat or tongue, swollen lips, wheezing, diarrhea, or vomiting—after eating certain foods, make an appointment with a doctor. (If your child is having trouble breathing, call emergency services.) Before the appointment, read "But She's Already Allergic" in chapter 2 (page 48), and consider printing out studies, such as those linked to on my website, to bring with you.

One to Three Years Old: The Most Difficult Feeding Phase

Here is where things get tricky. Your baby has become a toddler, and with her increased mobility, there is also increased intellectual prowess. While, yes, babies have their preferences, toddlers are downright opinionated. And unlike the baby, a toddler's opinions can shift dramatically even in the course of a day. The food that was loved last week is shunned today; the meal she gobbled up and asked for seconds yesterday is met with a begrudging "No thank you!" (We are still working on tone of voice at our table.) The food that she hasn't touched in weeks is suddenly declared her favorite.

This is exhausting and impossible to predict. It helps to keep in mind that this is a normal developmental stage. The toddler is practicing having opinions and practicing having some control. All you can do is offer. Forcing will just make her eating worse as she fights harder for a sense of control over herself.

Ellyn Satter, a registered dietician who has written several influential books on eating and feeding children, says, "When the joy goes out of eating, nutrition suffers." Toddlers have an innate ability to feed themselves and get the nourishment they need if regularly offered, in a structured way, the opportunities to do so. They may eat all carbs one day, and cozy up to proteins the next, or eat lots at one meal and only nibble at the next, but researchers have found that when given a buffet of *healthful* choices, small children tend to eat according to recommended guidelines over time.

I was reminded of this recently after a short trip where I inadvertently denied my children their favorite vegetables, keeping them satiated with the foods that I *knew* would be readily accepted, like pasta and sandwiches. You should have seen the broccoli consumption on our first day home! I even caught Grant eating arugula by the fistful right out of the fridge.

Parents should decide where and when meals happen, and what foods will be on offer, allowing children to decide how much, and whether, they eat those foods. Satter calls this the division of responsibility in feeding.

This is all fine and good, but what if you have good reason to worry about life-threatening allergies taking over your household? Can you just put the nut butter satay out on the table and say a little prayer to the allergy gods that your little one will magically partake? Isn't this a bit naive, especially for those kids who have a quite understandable aversion to a food for which they may be allergy prone?

This has definitely been the case in my house. And you can no longer spoon-feed a toddler. So how do you get them to take their allergen doses? How to do it nicely? Without driving yourself to the edge and without robbing your toddler of her growing sense of competency in paying attention to her own desires and appetites?

It is tricky. The main advice I have is to make the food really good. Pay attention to the tastes and textures your child likes best and then find ways to present the allergen in that format.

Going crispy is one popular way for this age group and it is good for a picky eater at any age. And it makes sense: If your body feels wary about a particular food, it is likely to be safest and thus most palatable if it has been well cooked. Crispiness is a way of

Don't force. *Tempt!*

signaling to the mouth and body that this is a well-cooked food. Even the pickiest eaters seem to agree on a few foods, nearly all of them crispy, such as well-cooked bacon, saltines, potato chips, and toasted white bread. In our house, we pan-fry salmon skin until it crackles like bacon, roast broccoli until it is charred and crunchy, and fry eggs over such a hot flame the bottoms crack with your first bite.

The other texture that seems universally popular is that of another well-cooked food: bread. Many allergens can be worked into a batter, whether it is using whole wheat flour, nut flours, seed butters, or extra eggs. Similarly, adding bread crumbs to fish can tone down the fishiness for the fish-averse child. Try mixing them with ground fish to make "fish burgers" or using them to coat strips of fish to make fish fingers (see page 207).

Attune yourself to your toddler's preferred tastes and textures; present allergens accordingly.

Shape still matters. During his entire toddlerhood, Grant would eat anything shaped like a stick or finger, from raw broccoli and peppers to a strategically cut burger. Some kids in this age group love the control, and creativity, that comes with having various dips to enjoy (or refuse).

And of course, the surefire way of making an allergen go down is presenting it as a dessert. Sugar can hide even the most off-putting flavors. When Dr. Lack told me to give Clara a daily slice of cake, we started having a designated dessert time each evening. I probably would have otherwise eschewed sweets for most of her toddlerhood, but it ended up being a blessing that went beyond fighting off her egg allergy. She never begs for sweets. If she or her brothers ask for something sweet at a different point in the day, they are met with knee-slapping laughter: "Oh ho, it is not dessert time!" And they don't fight it, as they've just been reminded, and assured, there *will* be a time for dessert.

Especially if you are using dessert to fight allergies, do not offer any other desserts or sweets at any other time in the day. You want sweets to be a truly special thing, something they get only once a day. You want them running to the dessert/allergen table in anticipation. Many of the recipes in this book hide major allergens amid a bit of sugar, flour, and butter. Try them, and wow, watch the allergens go down. In the most delightful way.

(And if one of you comes up with a fish dessert recipe, please share!)

Three to Five Years Old

By this point, preferences are a little less erratic, but it may still be hard to get your preschooler to eat allergens. Hopefully, especially if they've been eating them since they were babies, they will see them as friendly, yummy foods and you'll have no problems. But for some kids, as they get older, their food repertoire actually shrinks.

Again, trying to force them to eat will only backfire. Mealtimes need to be pleasant. No one wants to be cooperative and open to new experiences on a battleground.

Many of the strategies that worked when he was a toddler will continue to work at this age. Crispy or bready textures, fun shapes, creative dips, and desserts will remain popular. Clara is no longer allergic to eggs or nuts, but she won't touch them unless they are well hidden. And hide them I do, in pancakes, sandwiches, muffins, cookies, and other desserts, all to ensure that her allergies don't come back. Making sure the child sees you eating all the various foods at the table can also continue to help them feel the offending item is not only safe but, perhaps, even tasty.

The advantages of this age are the huge improvement in language abilities alongside their burgeoning curiosity in the way their bodies work. Unless they have somehow been taught that eating well is not cool, most kids have a natural interest in being healthy. They've experienced being ill and they know it is no fun. They may be boisterous and energetic, but they are aware of their own fragility (unlike teenagers). So with your preschooler, you can actually talk about health and about how what they eat affects their health. You can explain allergy prevention to them and explain, in simple language, how staying free of allergies will help them have more freedom in general as they get older. I still remember Clara's face when I explained that if her egg allergy came back, she wouldn't be able to get ice cream from an ice cream truck, like, ever. (Many types of ice cream have egg as an ingredient.) In went one of my Eggs Pretending to Be Muffins (page 111)!

> **Eat allergens yourself; if your child sees you enjoying a food, she is more likely to try and like it herself.**

The research is very young, but currently scientists at the forefront of the field believe that if allergens are eaten regularly for the first five years of life, most children will be well protected from developing an allergy from there on out. The regularity is important; intermittent exposure could allow an allergy to slip in between the cracks. In later childhood, first grade, and beyond, regularity may not be as necessary. One important study, LEAP-On, which was referenced in previous chapters, showed that if kids regularly ate peanuts for the first five years of life and then stopped completely, their tolerance to peanuts remained for at least one year. The researchers speculate that the tolerance will likely last indefinitely. That said, for several months, while I was finishing this book, I slipped to feeding five-year-old Clara egg only once a week—until one weekend she broke out in hives after eating her favorite, egg-soaked French toast. Back to twice a week we went! And her reactions subsided again. So, in my house, to play it safe, I will continue feeding my kids allergens twice a week until my youngest is through grade school.

The Complications of the Second (or Third or More) Kid

After Clara's allergies were diagnosed, I banned all the nuts Clara was allergic to from the house. To be honest, if I could have banned all almonds, cashews, pistachios, hazelnuts, Brazil nuts, macadamia nuts, and their associated products from the entire town, I would have. Like most, if not all, parents, my daughter's life is more precious to me than my popularity or anyone else's snacking pleasure. I wanted to preserve safety at all costs. I limited the entire household to the four nuts she could eat, the ones I faithfully gave her every day on Dr. Lack's orders.

> **Feed allergens to your baby when your allergic toddler is not around.**

Less than a week after Clara's second birthday, we welcomed her brother Grant to the family. When he was four months old, I took him to see Dr. Lack because I knew Grant was at an increased risk of developing allergies considering his sister's history. Luckily, despite his eczema, Grant's skin-prick tests indicated that no major allergies had yet developed. I initially felt relief. But then Dr. Lack explained that Grant was at risk for developing serious food allergies over the next couple years if I didn't act right then to protect him. Scribbling on his note pad, he commanded me to immediately and systematically introduce all major allergens, including each and every nut. He then explained that while it wasn't yet 100 percent conclusive, his hypotheses and research were pointing in the direction of early exposure to allergens, especially for those, like Grant, who are considered at high risk due to existing food allergies in a sibling.

I was stunned. I knew that even small amounts of most nuts had the potential to kill Clara, and here her doctor was telling me to feed them to her infant brother. Had he never seen siblings play with one another? Did he not understand that something you give to one is either going to be demanded by the other, or at the very least, smeared all over everyone in one way or another?

I voiced my concerns and Dr. Lack persevered. It had to be done. "Try to feed Grant when Clara isn't around," he suggested. But apart from the six hours a week she attended preschool, it seemed Clara was always around!

I did manage to do quite a bit while she was sleeping, making secret nut butters in the evening and labeling them aggressively. There was Grant's nut butter, with every nut blended in, including the six considered life threatening for his sister, and Clara's blend of four safe nuts. After making Grant's nut butter, with my heart pounding in my ears, I would scrub every surface and wash the food processor twice by hand before running it solo through the dishwasher. The sponges I used to clean with went into the trash and the rags were immediately run in the washing machine, so worried was I that Clara might come across them somehow. (As a toddler, she liked to "help" with the laundry.)

After an allergen feeding, be vigilant about cleaning up spit-ups and trace amounts on baby's hands, face, and hair.

In addition to the multiple labels, including ones that read DO NOT GIVE TO CLARA!, Grant's nut butter was put into a very different-looking container and had a plastic bag tied around it, so that even in the hazy tunnel of sleep deprivation (remember, Grant was only a few months old) and the rush to make Clara's nut butter sandwich, nobody could *ever* accidentally pull out the wrong jar.

I would feed baby Grant as a random daily snack *his* nut butter while Clara was at nursery school or taking a nap, and then immediately afterward I'd scrub down the kitchen and high chair (which is hard to do with a baby on your hip). I would then watch him closely for any spit-ups over the rest of the afternoon. Often he would smear some of the nut butter in his hair or spit up on my chest and then it would be baths and changes of clothes for one or both of us. It was a scary, exhausting time.

Fortunately, a couple months later, we had a much more reassuring visit with Dr. Lack. A new round of skin-prick testing for Clara showed a massive reduction in nearly all her allergies. A significant red welt still rose for almond, but everything else was minuscule. A few weeks later, again in Lack's office, we anxiously fed her cashews, ground up and mixed with a bit of yogurt, for the first time. We waited a couple hours and went home, in awe of how anticlimactic the visit was. She could now safely eat cashews and pistachios (which have similar allergic properties as cashews), and they were added to her usual daily nut butter. A week later, I gave her hazelnuts in a similar fashion and then Brazil and macadamia nuts.

For almonds, the worry over an anaphylactic reaction was considerably larger due to the persistent reaction in the skin-prick testing. So, to introduce almond for the first time, we went to a special hospital where she sat in a chair surrounded by other kids doing similar food challenges. The place was strewn with books, toys, and sealed plastic bags of allergens. Each child had a nurse closely monitoring them, along with a mother, father, or both and often a sibling or two in tow. The room was loud, bright, and saturated with a strange sharp boredom. There were EpiPens and defibrillators nearby. Everyone there was perched and waiting for an adverse, sudden event. Just waiting.

Clara, now two and a half years old, sat in a large cushioned medical chair, the type you might find at the dentist, enjoying the attention. I fed her a little bit of almond butter mixed with yogurt. And we waited about forty-five minutes. When nothing happened we fed her more, until she had eaten the ground equivalent of seven almonds. We waited several hours, watching her closely, fending off the boredom of herself and her infant brother. And then we went home profoundly relieved. Clara was allergy-free!

On Dr. Lack's orders, Grant was gradually introduced to egg also at four months, and although he didn't like it, I learned to hide it in puree and get it down him. He had some minor hives after eating egg as a baby, but by the time he was a toddler, I largely considered him allergy-free and didn't worry if he turned his nose up at the nuts and eggs I was continuing to be vigilant feeding Clara.

And then when he was two, the eczema on his scalp became more severe and the skin on other parts of his body started turning to sandpaper. My attention turned. He had recently started refusing nut butter sandwiches. When was the last time he had eaten egg? He refused to even try the eggy pancakes Clara loved, no matter how drowned they were in maple syrup. (I know, what kid doesn't like pancakes!) He also went off pasta, pizza, and grilled cheese sandwiches. He hadn't tasted fish since babyhood (not out of lack of my trying!). It seemed he subsisted on fruit, roasted broccoli, carrot sticks, oatmeal, and the occasional sausage—not a bad diet for a toddler, but really allergen poor.

It is normal for two-year-olds to get more opinionated, especially about what they eat. Grant's natural penchant for vegetables and fruit was, and is, wonderful, but was he eating enough of various allergens to be adequately protected? *Feeding multiple little children is always met with this challenge: They all like different things.* Usually I feel I've done well if there is at least one thing at the table *everyone* likes even if it is just a family-size tub of yogurt. But when it comes to allergens, I would need to be more hands on.

I wasn't too worried about wheat, as Grant still liked crackers. A lot. (This was before I knew that crackers aren't really protective; see "Wheat Allergy Prevention" in chapter 4 [page 92]. Luckily, whole wheat toast was still on his acceptable list.) So, for a while he got his dairy, egg, and fish doses strictly through cheese "crackers," salmon "crackers," and egg "crackers," which basically involved putting the allergen in a pan and shallow-frying it until it became crispy.

I did continue to visually expose him to allergens in more commonly eaten forms, remembering that kids need to see some foods at least a dozen times before they may be ready to try it. By "expose," I mean simply that I would put them on the table, eat them myself, and offer them to him. I never demanded that he taste something, and I never put anything in his mouth by force. Often the most effective trick was to physically hand a food to him. Grant seems almost unable to find the foods put on his plate, but if I put something into his hand, into his mouth it goes. Today, as a gravelly-voiced three-year-old, Grant still loves fruit and many vegetables, but he will also eat cold cheese slices, nuts in any form, hard-boiled eggs, fish—and, only sometimes, if I add Nutella, a bite or two of a pancake.

IN AN ALLERGY-FREE NUTSHELL

1. During pregnancy and lactation, there is no need to avoid allergenic foods.

2. Introduce all major allergens between three and five months of age if your baby is developmentally ready. Consult with a doctor first if your baby has dry skin, eczema, or a family history of allergies.

3. Work up to the suggested doses before your baby becomes six months old.

4. Keep a diary until feeding these doses becomes routine. The easiest route, at least in the beginning, may be to combine the allergens into one puree and give daily.

5. Tempt, rather than force, a toddler into eating his or her allergen dose.

6. Early, regular exposure to allergens may be safer than late or intermittent exposure.

Chapter 4

Prevention

To protect your baby from food allergy development, the best strategy, based on the most current science, is to introduce allergens early and continue feeding them to your child regularly, two or more times a week, for at least the first five years of his life. Ideally, this should be done for all major allergens, even if you are only worried about egg or nut allergy due to your particular family history. *Remember that food allergies are not completely explained by classical genetics and while you are busy protecting your son from peanut allergy, a wheat allergy could erupt or vice versa.* While many, but certainly not all, of the families I talked to described environmental allergies (e.g., hay fever) or other food allergies in their immediate or extended family, almost none had direct experience with the particular food allergy their child was exhibiting before seeing it in their child. "We are all pretty healthy; I have no idea where Ben's nut allergy came from," Pippa said, in what I soon realized would be a typical response, which should not be surprising considering the rate that food allergy prevalence is rising.

The ideal doses are still being worked out, but most likely, this is a case of "the more, the better." To provide at least some guidance, however, the EAT study asked parents to feed their babies (starting from three to four months old), toddlers, and preschoolers at least 2 grams of each allergen protein a week.

The amount of protein in each food varies, so please use the following charts for user-friendly allergen doses.

Weekly Guidelines for Preventing Food Allergies

- 2 1.5-ounce (40 g) containers plain yogurt or dairy equivalent (full fat for children under two years old)

- 1 small egg

- 3 rounded teaspoons peanut butter (use smooth, not chunky, for babies) or 5 teaspoons ground peanuts

- 3 teaspoons tahini or sesame equivalent

- 0.9 ounce (25 g) fish (about ¼ of an adult serving)

- 1 slice of whole wheat bread or wheat equivalent

If the amount of food seems daunting, take heart. It doesn't matter what form the various items are in; they can be pureed, baked in a cake, or stirred into a smoothie, as long as they go down. And remember, this is the *weekly* amount. Especially in the beginning, when you are dealing with the meager appetite of an infant, it can be helpful to break this down into five or even seven servings. By the time you have a toddler on your hands, the amounts will seem quite reasonable.

Cow's Milk Allergy Prevention

Cow's milk allergy is the most common food allergy in young children, affecting an estimated 2 percent of children under four years old. While some of the symptoms are the same, it should not be confused with lactose intolerance, a well-known but rare problem among young children.

In cow's milk allergy, the immune system mistakenly identifies milk proteins, such as casein and whey, as harmful. It then launches an attack, led by IgE, histamine, and other chemicals, leading to an allergic reaction. Cow's milk allergy may present with gas, diarrhea, and other gut issues, but it will also include immune-specific responses, such as rash, runny nose, cough, or wheezing.

Cow's milk allergy should not be confused with lactose intolerance.

Lactose intolerance, on the other hand, is when the digestive system simply can't digest the sugar, called lactose, in milk. The sugar then sticks around, feeding gut bacteria, giving rise to digestive issues similar to those in cow's milk allergy but without the immune-specific responses. Lactose intolerance is more prevalent among certain ethnic groups, including Asians, Hispanics, and people of African Caribbean descent. It has a very strong genetic component, and early exposure to dairy is unlikely to prevent it.

Cow's milk allergy, on the other hand, may be possible to avoid. To help prevent cow's milk allergy, introduce dairy, preferably as plain full-fat yogurt, when your baby is between three and four months old. After yogurt has been introduced, other milk products can be given to baby, such as cheese and cottage cheese. Whole cow's milk can also be given, but not as a drink for the first year of life, as it is nutritionally inferior to breast milk and formula. Instead, cook with it. Some ideas include:

- Use in place of water when making oatmeal.
- Dissolve wheat cereal in warm milk to make a wheat porridge.
- Add to potatoes or other vegetables before mashing.
- Poach fish in milk.
- Use to make a cheese sauce for pasta (see page 166).

The chart below shows different products that can help you meet the dairy dose. Choose one or divide and mix and match from different categories to meet the weekly dose. For example, you could give two 1.5-ounce containers of yogurt over a week's time or one 1.5-ounce container and ⅓ cup whole milk. Or make a small pizza with the recommended amount of mozzarella and serve half today, half tomorrow. If your child hates milk, yogurt, and cheese, turn to my pancake recipes and dairy desserts.

Try to meet the weekly dose, by whatever combination, by the time your baby is five months old. It is fine to exceed the amount so don't worry if, after you've met the required amount, your child wants significantly more.

Please note, to be nutritionally adequate, all dairy products should be full fat for children under two years old.

Dairy Product	Weekly Amount
Plain Yogurt*	2 1.5-ounce (40g) containers
Plain Thick-Style Greek Yogurt†	4 tablespoons (¼ cup); about 2 ounces (60 g)
Full-Fat Cottage Cheese	2 tablespoons (⅛ cup); about 1 ounce (30 g)
Whole Milk	⅔ cup (150 ml)
Mini Round Cheeses	2 round cheeses, together weighing 1.5 ounces (40 g)
Hard Cheeses	2 cubes, together weighing 0.5 ounce (16 g)
Processed Cheese Slices	About ⅔ a standard slice, weighing 0.5 ounce (16 g)
Mozzarella Ball	0.85 ounce (24 g)

*If using a multiserving container of plain full-fat yogurt, try for 7 or 8 large spoonfuls, or about a half cup, a week.

†Strained, thick-style Greek yogurt should have about 9 grams of protein per 100 grams. Runnier nonstrained varieties have half that amount and are comparable to regular yogurts. If using a multiserving container of nonstrained Greek yogurt, with around 4.5 grams of protein per 100 grams, aim for 7 or 8 large spoonfuls a week.

Egg Allergy Prevention

The recommended guideline for prevention of egg allergy is to feed your baby and child at least one egg a week. This should be broken down into two or more servings over the course of a week's meals.

Young children need extra protection from sicknesses such as salmonella poisoning. Be sure to buy high-quality fresh eggs and consider pasteurized eggs, such as Davidson's Safest Choice. (They now have cage-free eggs for us free-range enthusiasts.) Always cook eggs thoroughly, and when serving leftovers, reheat thoroughly before serving, even if your toddler prefers everything room temp. She'll just have to wait until they cool down again; killing any bacteria that could have multiplied during storage is most important.

For many adults, fried eggs, toast, and bacon are the epitome of comfort food. But eggs can have an unpleasant taste for some babies and children.

> **Ensure your child eats at least one small egg a week from three and a half months old until at least age five.**

To start your baby off, the surest bet is to make a puree of hard-boiled eggs. This ensures the egg is fully cooked and it can be relatively easy to hide the egg taste in a puree of other yummy food, such as peas, avocado, potatoes, or fruit. Make the puree in bulk, freeze some, and portion doses out over several meals, making sure you reach the equivalent of a full egg by the end of the week.

Scrambled eggs, especially with small soft curds (see page 107), are also a good option, especially if your baby seems to like egg flavor. However, some parents, including myself, see their babies react to scrambled eggs, with hives and the like, while the baby seems to have no problem with hard-boiled or baked eggs. It is possible that when egg is cooked more thoroughly, at a higher temperature, the protein changes, making it less likely to trigger an allergic reaction.

In general, it is best for small children and babies to avoid raw and undercooked egg, such as that found in hollandaise sauce, homemade mayonnaise, soft meringue, or any cake where the batter hasn't fully set.

Nut Allergy Prevention Guidelines

For most babies, peanuts should be introduced when the infant is between three and four months old. Use a full-fat smooth peanut butter, with at least 95 percent peanut content in the ingredient list, or see my primer on making your own nut butter on page 133. Mix into purees or yogurt, or thin it with breast milk or formula. In infancy, it may be easiest to give a small amount every day, so by the end of the week you can be confident that your baby has met the 3-teaspoon quota.

Introduce peanut butter at three months of age—checking with your allergist first, if you have a high-risk baby.

For the older baby and beyond, you can sub in finely ground plain peanuts. You can stir these into purees or use it as flour for baked goods—a great way to mask the taste if your little one is peanut averse. Please see the nut recipe chapter for more ways to present peanuts in child-friendly forms.

It is best to *steer clear of chunky peanut butter until one year of age* to minimize choking risk. In toddlerhood, full-fat crunchy peanut butter can be used. Again, make sure it has at least 95 percent peanut content or contains at least 25 grams of protein per 100 grams of product. This information is usually readily available on the nutrition label. Most natural peanut butters provide the required amount of peanut content and protein, but if your child prefers a more processed taste, choose Skippy over Jif. Smooth Skippy peanut butter has 25.3 grams of protein per 100 grams of butter; Jif only has 21.9 grams. That said, Skippy's peanut content is only 90 percent, due to the addition of sugar and palm oil, so if you can switch to a natural peanut butter, and have your child still eat it readily, do!

Peanut	Weekly Amount
Smooth Peanut Butter	3 rounded teaspoons (at least 16 g)
Finely Ground Peanuts	5 level teaspoons (16 g)
Crunchy Peanut Butter (from one year old)	3 rounded teaspoons (at least 16 g)

Research is still mounting for other nuts, with critical studies in progress when this book went to press. It is expected that what seems to be working for peanuts and likely other major allergens will also work for tree nuts: To help protect your child from tree nut allergy, feed them to your baby early, carefully, and often. If your baby is considered high risk, have him tested first for existing nut allergies. The theory of early exposure suggests it is best to introduce as early as possible, ideally between three and six months, assuming the baby is healthy and developmentally ready to eat solids (i.e., she can hold her head up and seems interested in food).

Introduce each nut in some type of ground form, such as a nut butter or nut flour. You may want to mix it with water, breast milk, or runny plain yogurt. After introduction, twice weekly exposure to all nuts is likely necessary, for at least the first five years of life. This requires a tremendous amount of organization and work. To simplify my own life, and yet keep my children nut-allergy free, I make a nut butter combining all nuts (see page 133.) I usually make this in bulk, six or seven jars' worth, and then freeze them for use over the next several months. In addition to using the recipes in the nut section of this book, I spread the mixed-nut butter on crackers for an afterschool snack every weekday. This routine helps me feel confident that my kids are getting enough nut exposure without the stress of trying to remember the last time Grady had macadamia nuts and Arthur had pecans.

Unfortunately, the exact amount a baby or child needs to consume of each tree nut is currently unknown and will likely vary for each nut. Estimated weekly doses for all allergens are currently set to provide about 2 grams of protein content. Peanuts have more protein per serving than other nuts (in some cases, quite a bit more; see the chart below). Therefore, it is expected that higher doses of other nuts may be required to protect children from various tree nut allergies. That said, there could be compounding properties. For example, eating pistachios may protect from both cashew and pistachio allergy. We'll have to stay tuned. For now, I tell myself, some is better than none and continue to give my children mixed-nut butter on a near daily basis.

Shelled Nut	Protein Content per 100 Grams of Nut	Protein Content per 25-Gram Serving
Peanuts	26.2 g	6.6 g
Almonds	21.2 g	5.3 g
Cashews	18.2 g	4.6 g
Pistachios	17.9 g	4.5 g
Walnuts	15.2 g	3.8 g
Hazelnuts	15.0 g	3.7 g
Brazil Nuts	14.3 g	3.6 g
Pine Nuts	13.7 g	3.4 g

Shelled Nut	Protein Content per 100 Grams of Nut	Protein Content per 25-Gram Serving
Pecans	10.9 g	2.7 g
Macadamia Nuts	7.9 g	2.0 g

Sesame Allergy Prevention

Sesame allergy is a growing problem, and sufferers are plagued by the fact that sesames, or traces of sesame, can be found in the most innocuous places, from pizza crust, to margarine, even lip balm. To try to protect your baby from this allergy, it will likely be easiest to start with tahini, a Middle Eastern staple, which is usually nothing more than ground sesame seeds. Often the oil rises to the top in a jar or tin of tahini; simply mix it back in before serving. Tahini can taste a bit bitter, so mixing it into smooth palatable foods can be helpful. For babies, mix tahini into breast milk, plain full-fat yogurt, mashed sweet potatoes or bananas, or rice porridge. "Light" tahini can be used as long as it contains at least 26 grams of protein per 100 grams of tahini. This should be clear from the nutritional label.

> Ground sesame is naturally bitter.
> Mix with something palatable, like
> bananas or potatoes.

You can also use full-fat hummus, which is basically tahini with chickpeas blended in. A teething baby may find hummus on a cold cucumber stick particularly delightful. Hummus is also yummy, even to toddlers and preschoolers, spread on a plain rice cake, toast, crudités, even apple slices. Try my Rainbow Hummus (page 159) and let your kids get creative decorating rice cakes, cucumber circles, or my Savory Falafel "Cookies" (page 154) with different colors of hummus.

Sesame seeds can also be used in home-baked goods or stirred whole into yogurts, oatmeal, and rice. A couple teaspoons scattered over noodles or sticky chicken drumsticks can be delicious and fun. (Let the toddler do the scattering!) Just make sure to measure first, so that you know how much to count each serving toward the weekly protective dose.

Sesame seeds found on store-bought breadsticks, crackers, rolls, and so on are fine for kids to eat, but do not count them toward the weekly required amount of sesame. The amount of sesame on these products is rarely enough to make a significant contribution to the required dose. That said, if you'd like to make similar products at home, carefully measuring the amount of sesame used (and eaten), then they could be used to meet the weekly dose.

Sesame	Weekly Amount
Tahini	3 teaspoons (15 g)
Hummus*	About 8 rounded tablespoons (120 g)
Sesame Seeds	About 8 heaped teaspoons (22 g)

*Make sure the hummus ingredient list includes tahini or sesame.

Fish Allergy Prevention

At about four months old, introduce your infant to fish. Start off with white fish, such as cod or haddock, and work the baby up to eating 25 grams, or about a quarter of the average fillet, on a weekly basis. Again, mixing fish with other palatable foods, such as breast milk, avocados, and potatoes, can help ensure the baby is receptive. Be careful to remove any and all bones.

Once your baby is five months old, you can start giving him oily fish, such as salmon and trout, as well. Variety is a good sign of a healthful diet, even for a baby. Avoid, however, fish types that are known to be high in mercury, such as swordfish. Mercury can cause serious health problems, and young developing brains are considered particularly at risk. See the lists on page 92 for examples of acceptable, and unacceptable, fish choices.

One note: Tuna, a childhood favorite, is particularly complicated when it comes to mercury. In general, bigger fishes are further down the food chain and have greater concentrations of mercury in their flesh. So the trick to avoiding mercury is to avoid big fishes. Well, just to trip us up, tuna comes in different sizes. For canned tuna, you either have big albacore tuna or "white tuna" or smaller skipjack tuna for "light tuna." According to the Environmental Defense Fund, children under six should not eat more than one 3-ounce serving of white tuna in any given month and not more than three 3-ounce servings of light tuna in a month.

A further note about canned fish: Canned fish will have more salt content than frozen or fresh fish. Choosing the kind packed in water or oil will have less salt than those packed in brine or tomato sauce. Cans also come with worries about BPA, a compound that, in large amounts, has been linked to a wide range of health problems, possibly due to its hormone-mimicking properties.

Cooking fresh fish can be a lot easier than we sometimes think. Simply put a fish fillet on an oiled baking sheet and put the baking sheet in a warm oven (say, 375°F). Take it out when it is cooked through, usually 10 to 15 minutes. Done.

Fish	Weekly Amount
Fresh/Frozen Fish	¼ 3.5-ounce fillet (about 25 g)
Fish Sticks	2 average fish sticks
Canned Fish	About 0.8 ounces (25 g), drained

Types of Fish to Embrace		Types of Fish to Avoid
White Fish	**Oily**	Shark
Cod	Salmon	Marlin
Flounder	Mackerel	Swordfish
Sole	Herring	White/Albacore Tuna
Pollack	Pilchard	(not more than once a
Haddock	Sardine	month)
Plaice	Trout	

What About Shellfish?

It is expected that early exposure to shellfish will help protect against the development of shellfish allergy later in life. However, there have not yet been studies directly assessing this. The majority of shellfish allergy sufferers experience their first reaction as adults; shellfish allergy in infancy is very unlikely, and giving shellfish to babies may protect them long term.

Cold jumbo shrimp was one of Arthur's favorites when he first started teething. Canned crabmeat, mixed with a bit of tomato paste, can make an excellent pasta sauce. I've also included ground shrimp in my salmon sliders (see page 205), to protect my kids from fish and shellfish allergy simultaneously.

Wheat Allergy Prevention

Of the parents I talked to, the ones who had children who could not eat wheat were those who suffered most. Wheat is everywhere—and for most kids, immensely palatable. (That said, as a child with undiagnosed celiac disease, I detested sandwiches and cereal.) I don't know many adults who will happily shun a piece of cake, let alone hyped-up children at a birthday party. To say nothing about other childhood staples, such as crackers, sandwiches, pretzels, cookies, and pizza. And then there are all of wheat's hiding places! Wheat can lurk in ice cream, yogurt, sauces, sausages, and even chocolate, just to name a few. Parents with wheat-allergic children not only have to protect their children from all these temptations but also deal with the sense of deprivation and isolation that many of these children feel.

Wheat allergy should not be confused with celiac disease or wheat intolerance.

So it is not surprising, therefore, that many parents want to keep this allergy from developing in the first place. To protect your child, it may be helpful to introduce wheat between four to five months of age and then offer it biweekly for the first five years of life. You may want to avoid introducing wheat before four months because there are some concerns that it will promote celiac disease. That said, some scientists think these concerns are misguided.

It is important that the wheat consumed is whole grain wheat, not items made from overprocessed "white" flours, such as most crackers, cakes, cookies, and white bread. The latter can be eaten as well, but it is unlikely to be very protective. Whole grain wheat products have significant amounts of protein which is thought to enable these products to teach the immune system about wheat's safety. Similarly, if using pasta or couscous to meet the required dose (see table on page 94), be sure to use products that are made of 100 percent wheat. That is, pastas that include egg, and couscous that includes other grains or ingredients, should not be counted toward the weekly wheat dose.

In the United Kingdom, where the EAT study was conducted, Weetabix is an extremely popular cereal for both children and adults, and thus it was relied upon heavily within the study. It comes in both large and small "biscuits," similar in size to large and small Shredded Wheat but with a texture more closely resembling a crumbly version of Wheat Chex. Many major grocery stores in the United States carry Weetabix, but you might have to spend some time scouring the cereal aisle or searching Amazon and other online retailers before finding it. Snatch it up if you can; kids and babies love it, and it lends itself easily to various yummy baked goods (see "Recipes for Wheat Allergy Prevention" on page 182). Fortunately, a U.S. favorite, Wheat Chex will also provide adequate amounts of wheat protein to protect from wheat allergy, but your child will have to eat slightly more of the cereal to meet the required dose. Remember that the dose is best divided into at least two feedings over the course of a week. Eating more than the required dose, even significantly more, is fine. From an allergy-prevention perspective, the more exposure, the better.

Wheat	Weekly Amount
Weetabix, Large	2 biscuits
Weetabix, Bite Size	⅔ cup
Wheat Chex	¾ cup
Plain Whole Wheat Bread, Thin Slices	2 slices
Plain Whole Wheat Bread, Thick Slices	½ slice
Plain Whole Wheat Pita Bread	1 6-inch pita, weighing 1.75 ounces (50 g)
Pasta or Couscous (100% wheat)	1.5 ounces or 40 grams, uncooked (see below)
Pasta	Weekly Amount (40 grams, uncooked)
Macaroni	½ cup
Spaghetti	44 sticks
Fusilli	½ cup
Couscous	¼ cup

It is important to note that wheat allergy is different from celiac disease and wheat intolerance. True wheat allergy has all the hallmark symptoms of a proper allergy: itchy or runny nose, rash or hives, swelling, wheezing or asthma, and in some cases, anaphylaxis. There can also be stomach pain and loose stools.

While there is evidence that some wheat allergy symptoms can be delayed by twenty-four to forty-eight hours, usually the symptoms are immediate or near immediate upon ingesting or coming in contact with wheat.

Celiac disease is also characterized by an erroneous immune response, one to a protein within wheat, rye, and barley called gluten. But in celiac disease, a different cascade of reactions is in play, separate from the IgE reactions typical of a classic food allergy. The symptoms of celiac disease tend to be more delayed and largely gastrointestinal. Unchecked, it can also lead to inadequate nutrition, giving rise to poor growth rates and other problems.

Wheat intolerance is a poorly understood problem that causes gastrointestinal distress and fatigue, but is unlikely to be life threatening. It is not thought to directly involve the immune system.

Avoidance of gluten has become popular in many circles as people have associated it to a broad array of health problems, from irritable bowel syndrome and limb numbness to depression and weight gain. Some people, thought to be suffering from nonceliac gluten sensitivity, see improvements in their symptoms when they cut gluten from their diet.

Early exposure to wheat will likely protect a child from wheat allergy, but so far the data are inconclusive that it will help ward off other problems with wheat and gluten.

Prevention of Soy, Kiwi, and Other Allergies

The prevalence of allergies to kiwi, banana, soy, shellfish, and other foods are also most likely growing. There are some studies looking at tactics to desensitize and prevent some of these food allergies, but few have been conclusively finished. One or more of these allergens could be a complete outlier that does not fit the

....

Priming the immune system with a wide
variety of foods, especially common
allergens, could give lifelong protection
from food allergies.

....

overall pattern. That is, it could turn out that early exposure to say, soy, is not protective.

However, the overall approach—expose early and often—may prove to protect against most food allergies. The immune system is more likely to "trust" foods that it has come in contact with during infancy. We have proof of this *concept*, even if we do not yet have data on every single allergen. So with this caveat, there is enough evidence to encourage early exposure to shellfish, soy, kiwi, and any other foods of concern.

As there are no guidelines addressing these foods, just aim for regular exposure. Personally, without any sense of what might be the "right" amount or form, I give my kids fresh kiwi and bananas at least once a week and soy, in the form of edamame, twice a month. I am trying to get more shellfish into their diet, but currently they only eat it about once a month, usually with some bready coating.

IN AN ALLERGY-FREE NUTSHELL

1. Aim to protect your baby from all food allergies, even if there is only one type prevalent in your family history.

2. Introduce peanut, wheat, egg, dairy, sesame, and fish to your baby well before he reaches six months old. Consult with a doctor first if your baby has dry skin, eczema, or a family history of allergies.

3. You may also want to introduce other common food allergens, such as tree nuts, kiwi, banana, soy, and shellfish by the end of the fifth month.

4. Research is ongoing, but for now babies (starting from four months old), toddlers, and preschoolers should aim to eat at least 2 grams of each allergen protein a week. See the charts in this chapter for guidance.

5. Lactose intolerance, wheat intolerance, and celiac disease are not food *allergies*.

Chapter 5

Recipes

Countdown of Top Allergy-Preventing Recipes and Meal Ideas

All the recipes in this book aim to prevent the development of food allergies, but as a parent, I have found the ones that target multiple allergens at once to be the most convenient.

Below is a list of these powerhouse, multitasking recipes that combine multiple allergens into one yummy meal. I've listed them here for convenience, as each is only included once in the chapters beyond. That is, Sunrise Yogurt is found in the dairy chapter, although it will help prevent both egg and dairy allergies. Similarly, Nutty Noodles is found just once, in the chapter focusing on nuts, although it will help prevent egg, peanut, tree nut, sesame, wheat, and fish allergies. So if you can't find a recipe little Emma likes in the egg chapter, it is worth perusing this list to see egg-allergy-fighting recipes that have been included in other chapters. Use the icons detailed in the legend below to skim for recipes that offer protection from specific food allergies.

🥚 Egg 🥜 Peanut 🌰 Tree nut ⚫ Sesame 🥛 Dairy

🌾 Wheat 🐟 Fish ☀ Kiwi 🦐 Shellfish

Among the recipes are the nineteen used in the EAT study. These are denoted by the symbol *Eat*.

TWO ALLERGENS IN ONE MEAL

Sesame Fish Fingers, page 156

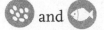 and

Sunrise Yogurt, page 165

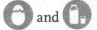 and

Cheese Balloon, page 114

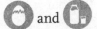 and

Faux-Fried Cheese Fingers, page 171

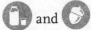 and , or

Yogurt Oatmeal Cookies made with nut flour, page 178

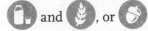 and

Sesame Cookies, page 193

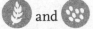 and

Neat Wheat Sliders or Meat "Breadsticks," page 187

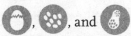 and

THREE ALLERGENS IN ONE MEAL

Egg, Tahini, and Peanut Butter Puree, page 106

, , and

Peanut-Tahini Dip or Sauce tossed with pasta, page 131

, , and

Eggy Cheese Soldiers, page 170

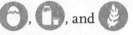

Cheese Balloon spread on whole wheat toast, page 114

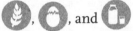

Weetabix Banana Muffins, page 185

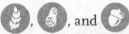

Weetabix Peanut Butter Chocolate Chip Cookies, page 191

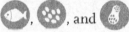

Nutty Fish Puree or Spread, page 200

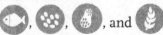

Tuna Bolognese, page 211

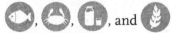

FOUR ALLERGENS IN ONE MEAL

Nutty Fish Puree or Spread served on whole wheat bread, page 200

Salmon-Shrimp Sliders topped with Greek yogurt and tucked in a whole wheat bun, page 205

Egg, Tahini, and Peanut Butter Puree with added tree nut butter, page 106

Peanut-Tahini Dip or Sauce made with added tree nut butter and tossed with pasta, page 131

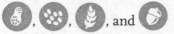

Time-Crunch Fish Sticks made with nut flour (page 207) alongside couscous and **Tahini-Honey Dip** (page 160) or Greek yogurt thinned with orange juice

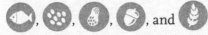

FIVE ALLERGENS IN ONE MEAL

Nutty Fish Puree or Spread made with mixed-nut butter, served on whole wheat bread, page 200

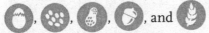

Egg, Tahini, and Mixed-Nut Butter Puree mixed or served with couscous, page 106

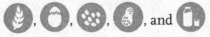

Wheaty Porridge Jambalaya, page 183

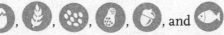

SIX ALLERGENS IN ONE MEAL

Nutty Noodles, page 141

EAT Wheaty Mix & Mash, page 201

WINNERS TAKE ALL:
NINE ALLERGENS IN ONE MEAL

For babies: **Kiwi EAT Wheaty Mix & Mash** (variation of recipe) with mixed-nut butter and shrimp blended in, page 202

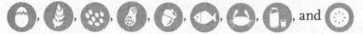, and ⊕

For toddlers and preschoolers: **Nutty Noodles** served with shrimp, a glass of milk, and sliced kiwi, page 141

◐, ◑, ◐, ◐, ◐, ◐, ◐, ◐, and ◑

Recipes for Egg Allergy Prevention

The weekly doses in these recipes are the *minimum* a baby or child is currently advised to eat. It is fine, perhaps even desirable, to surpass the required amounts. Try to offer each allergen at least twice a week, no matter the amount eaten the first day. So if your child wolfs down 1 egg on Monday, you still need to make sure she eats at least ⅓ an egg later in the week. The more egg your child eats, the better, from an allergy-prevention perspective.

Feed your baby and child at least one small egg every week.

EGGS FOR BABY

GREEN EGGS PUREE

I always think of the popular Dr. Seuss book *Green Eggs and Ham* when I make this. The sweetness of the pear makes the puree a treat going down. I could almost see baby Arthur thinking, "Say! I do like green eggs sans ham! Thank you, Mom-I-am!"

Makes 28.4 ounces (840 ml), or 14 2-ounce (60 ml) servings. One serving provides ½ weekly egg dose.

7 small hard-boiled eggs
2 ripe avocados, halved, pitted, and peeled
1 ripe pear, cored and seeded

1. Place all the ingredients in a blender and puree to desired smoothness.

2. Use two servings within the first 2 to 3 days of making. Freeze the remaining servings in 2-ounce (60 ml) baby food containers to use within the next few months. (Look for Stage 2 baby food containers through Amazon or a baby-focused retailer.) For older babies, who are ready to be challenged with textures beyond soupy smooth, serve with couscous or lumpy mashed potatoes.

Eat TAHINI-EGG SURPRISE

Tahini is so popular in Middle Eastern dishes, including the now globally popular hummus dip. My favorite is baba ganoush, a dip that combines grilled eggplant with tahini. I was tempted to name this recipe Eggy-Ganoush, but the above is more straightforward.

Makes about ½ cup. The full recipe provides the weekly sesame and egg doses, best served over 2 or more days.

1 small hard-boiled egg
2 tablespoons water
3 teaspoons tahini, well stirred
1 to 4 tablespoons boiling water

1. Place the egg and water in a blender and puree until it resembles a smooth paste. Add the tahini and boiling water and pulse until the mixture is the consistency your baby is most likely to prefer.

2. Store leftovers in an airtight container in the refrigerator for up to 2 days. Alternatively, make in bulk and freeze in individual portions for use over the next month. Defrost for several hours in the fridge and then reheat thoroughly in the microwave before serving.

Eat EGG, TAHINI, AND PEANUT BUTTER PUREE

This puree not only smells good (I love peanut butter), but it protects a baby from three allergens all in one go. A great multitasking recipe that can be served to baby with a spoon or, for toddlers or babies that are teething, spread on toast or rice cakes. You could also add a couple teaspoons of homemade tree nut butter (see page 133) to help protect from tree nut allergies simultaneously.

Makes about ⅔ cup.
The full recipe provides the weekly egg, sesame, and
peanut doses, best served over 2 or more days.

1 small hard-boiled egg
2 to 3 tablespoons water
3 teaspoons tahini, well stirred
3 rounded teaspoons smooth peanut butter
1 to 4 tablespoons boiling water

1. Place the egg and water in a blender and puree until it resembles a smooth paste. Add the tahini and blend. Thin out the peanut butter with 1 teaspoon boiling water and then add to the egg-tahini mixture and blend. Slowly add additional hot water, blending, until the mixture is the consistency your baby is most likely to prefer.

2. Store leftovers in an airtight container in the refrigerator for up to 2 days. Alternatively, make in bulk and freeze in individual portions for use over the next month. Defrost for several hours in the fridge and then reheat thoroughly in the microwave before serving.

BREAKFAST

SMALL CURD EGGS

If hard-boiled and baked eggs are well tolerated and liked, you can try offering your baby these well-cooked scrambled eggs. Keep the curds small and baby friendly by moving your spatula through the egg mixture the entire cooking time. Older kids and adults like these, too, so I usually quadruple the recipe and feed the whole family. My husband adores them on toast.

Makes about ⅛ cup.
The full recipe provides the weekly egg dose, best served over 2 or more days. This recipe also provides ½ dairy dose.
If you pair each serving with 2 tablespoons plain full-fat yogurt, you'll meet both egg and dairy weekly requirements.

  1 small egg
  2 tablespoons milk (use whole, especially if cooking for
    children under two)
  1 teaspoon unsalted butter

1. In a small bowl, beat the egg with the milk. Melt the butter in a small sauté pan over the lowest heat that your stovetop is capable of maintaining. Add the egg mixture and cook over low heat, stirring constantly for about 3 minutes, until thoroughly cooked through.

2. Store leftovers in an airtight container in the refrigerator for 3 to 4 days. Unfortunately, this dish does not freeze well.

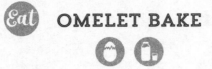 OMELET BAKE

Another recipe the whole family will love. Even better, it is incredibly flexible. Options for fillings and seasonings (if your kids like them) are limited only by your imagination. And it can be prepared, up to the baking step, 2 days in advance. If we are having weekend guests, I love to prepare this on Friday morning, tripling the recipe. I then store it in the fridge, covered with plastic wrap, while we entertain Friday night and Saturday. Sunday morning it gets popped into a hot oven for an easy-peasy brunch.

Makes about three ¾-cup servings. This freezable recipe provides 3 weekly egg doses and 1½ weekly dairy doses.

3 small eggs
3 tablespoons whole milk
3 tablespoons grated cheddar cheese
1 cup chopped or minced filling, such as ham, tuna, onions, peppers, tomatoes, sweet corn, or spinach, or a combination (optional)
1 to 2 teaspoons seasonings, such as sweet smoked paprika, black pepper, garlic, or mixed dried herbs

1. Preheat the oven to 350°F.

2. In a medium bowl, beat together the eggs and milk. Stir in the cheese and, if using, the filling with seasonings. Pour the mixture into a greased 8 × 8-inch casserole dish and bake for 20 to 30 minutes, until well set. You should be able to place a knife in the middle and have it come out clean, not gooey.

3. Store leftovers in an airtight container in the refrigerator for 3 to 4 days. Alternatively, portion it into weekly servings, wrap each individually, and store in the freezer for up to 2 months. Defrost for several hours in the fridge before using. Reheat in a microwave or in a 200°F oven until piping hot.

FRENCH TOAST

My daughter declared these "scrummy yummy" and rubbed her belly the first time I served these. Any bread will work, but baguettes easily provide small crusty pieces for small hands. I usually serve with fruit and Greek yogurt. You can also use regular sandwich bread, but after frying, toast in the oven for an extra 5 to 10 minutes. If you choose whole grain bread you can get a wheat dose in, too! I have also found these to be great for a teething baby; just leave the honey out and the toppings off—although a smear of nut butter might be nice!

Note: Honey may contain bacteria that can't be handled by the digestive system of a child less than one year old, so recipes containing honey should not be served to babies.

**Makes 16 small whole grain baguette slices:
4 slices contain ½ egg and 1 wheat dose. Or 3 whole grain
sandwich-bread-size slices: each slice has ⅓ egg and
1 weekly wheat dose. Serve twice over the week to
provide the weekly egg and wheat doses. Each serving
also provides about ¼ of the weekly dairy dose.**

2 small eggs
½ cup whole milk
¼ teaspoon vanilla extract
1 tablespoon honey (optional)
⅛ teaspoon ground cinnamon (optional)
1 small whole grain baguette, about 8 inches long, cut into
    ½-inch slices, or 3 slices whole grain sandwich bread
1 tablespoon butter

1. In a medium bowl, beat together the eggs, milk, vanilla, and, if using, the honey and cinnamon. This can be made a full day in advance and kept in an airtight container in the refrigerator until you are ready to make the toast.

2. Pour the egg mixture into a 9-inch pie pan. Soak the bread in the mixture, flipping once, until it is completely saturated and nearly all the liquid is gone. Melt the butter in a large skillet or griddle over medium heat and fry the bread until golden brown and crispy, about 3 minutes on the first side, and 2 on the other. If you like soft centers, serve immediately. If you (or your kids) prefer it crispy, after frying, bake the egg-soaked bread on a lightly greased baking sheet in a 400°F oven for 15 to 20 minutes, turning the slices once halfway through. I find this also helps me keep the toast hot, while I make more batches, allowing me to serve multiple people at once.

3. Topping ideas include butter, maple syrup, chocolate syrup, whipped cream, caramelized bananas, confectioners' sugar, brown sugar, Nutella, honey-nut butter (nut butter mixed with a generous amount of honey) or honey-yogurt sauce (Greek yogurt thinned with orange juice and sweetened with honey to taste).

4. Store leftovers in an airtight container in the refrigerator for 3 to 4 days. Alternatively, double or triple the recipe, portion it into weekly servings, wrap each individually in plastic wrap or sealable plastic storage bags, and store in the freezer for up to 2 months. Defrost in the fridge for 3 hours or at room temperature for about 50 minutes before using. Reheat in a 200°F oven until piping hot.

EGGS PRETENDING TO BE MUFFINS

Eggs disguised as baked goods. Need I say more?

**Makes 12 "muffins." Each muffin contains ¾ egg.
One and a half muffins, served over the course
of a week, provide the weekly egg dose.**

9 small eggs
¼ cup whole milk
⅓ cup all-purpose flour
¼ teaspoon baking soda
⅓ cup sugar
¼ teaspoon vanilla extract
⅛ teaspoon salt

1. Preheat the oven to 350°F. Lightly grease a 12-cup muffin pan and set aside.

2. In a medium bowl, beat together the eggs and milk. Add the flour, baking soda, sugar, vanilla, and salt, mixing well. Pour the batter into the pan and bake for 25 to 30 minutes, until golden brown and enormously puffy. These will collapse into pretty little muffins upon removing from the oven.

3. You can make this batter up to 2 days in advance and store in an airtight container in the refrigerator. The muffins taste best right out of the oven but are also good cold and great for packed lunches. Store leftovers in an airtight container in the refrigerator for up to 3 days, or freeze for up to 2 months. Defrost in the fridge and then reheat in the microwave or a 200°F oven until piping hot.

VARIATION: Go savory by leaving out the sugar and adding ½ cup chopped tomato, cooked broccoli, ham, crumbled sausage, or grated cheese.

EGGY BRUNCH PANCAKES

This is Clara's absolute favorite way to get her egg. Even baby Arthur, once he started cutting teeth, got in on the action. Small ones can be great for smaller hands, although large ones are enjoyed by preschoolers keen on showing off their knife skills. Cutting them into various geometric shapes is particularly popular in our house.

Makes 12 large pancakes. Each pancake has ¾ egg. One and a half pancakes, served over 2 different days, provide the weekly egg dose. Two and a half pancakes provide about ½ the weekly dairy dose.

9 small eggs
1½ cups milk
3 tablespoons butter, melted
3 tablespoons sugar
¾ teaspoon salt
¾ teaspoon vanilla extract (optional)
1¾ cups all-purpose flour
1 teaspoon baking soda
2 teaspoons cold butter
Pure maple syrup

1. In a large bowl, beat together the eggs and milk. Add the melted butter, sugar, salt, and, if using, the vanilla. Mix well. Stir in the flour and baking soda.

2. Preheat the oven to 175°F.

3. Heat the cold butter on a large griddle or frying pan over medium-high heat. Use a paper towel to gently wipe the butter around, evenly coating the pan's surface. (This will ensure that even your first pancake is pretty.)

4. Pour or scoop the batter onto the griddle, using approximately ⅓ cup for each pancake. When you see little bubbles forming in the batter, flip the pancake and cook until browned, about another minute or so. Place on a baking sheet and keep warm in the oven until all the pancakes are done. Serve with a drizzle of maple syrup on top.

5. The batter can be made a full day in advance and stored in the refrigerator. Store leftovers in an airtight container in the refrigerator for up to 4 days. They are best eaten warm. The pancakes can also be frozen for up to 2 months. Defrost fully at room temperature for a couple hours or overnight in the fridge before using. To reheat, warm them one by one in the microwave or spread them out onto baking sheets and place in a 200°F oven for 10 to 15 minutes. Don't stack them because they can stick to one another.

ADDITIONAL SERVING IDEAS (BEYOND MAPLE SYRUP):

- Nutella and banana: Spread a thin layer of Nutella over the slightly cooled pancake and let your toddler or preschooler "decorate" it with slices of banana.
- Whipped cream and strawberries: Make a face with strawberries for the eyes and nose, and a big whipped-cream smile.

LUNCH/DINNER

CHEESE BALLOON
(BETTER KNOWN AS SOUFFLÉ)

Soufflés really aren't as hard to make as they are reputed to be. And kids love watching soufflés rise. This soufflé comes to the table looking like a giant cheese balloon ready to be "popped" at the table by the first prick. And indeed, the rapid deflation is just as exciting.

Many young children are sensitive to heat, so serve individual portions with a plain yogurt, ketchup, or other cool sauce. Or let children spread some soufflé on toast; by the time they've finished spreading, the soufflé should be cool enough.

TIP: To separate egg whites from egg yolks, crack the egg over a wide bowl, and pass the egg yolk between the two halves of shell, letting the white fall into the bowl. It is easiest, but not essential, to do this when the eggs are at room temperature.

> Makes eight ½-cup child-size servings, or enough to feed 2 adults and 2 children. One-eighth of this recipe provides ½ weekly egg dose and 1 weekly dairy dose.

4 small eggs
¼ cup all-purpose flour
¼ teaspoon salt
1 cup whole milk
¾ cup (packed) shredded mild cheddar cheese
½ teaspoon cream of tartar

1. Preheat the oven to 350°F. Separate the eggs, placing the whites in a medium bowl and the yolks in a small bowl, and set aside. Allow the egg whites to warm to room temperature.

2. Mix the flour and salt in an unheated saucepan and gradually whisk in the milk until smooth. Place the pan over medium-high heat, and stirring constantly, cook the mixture until it thickens and boils. Turn off the heat and immediately add the cheese, stirring until melted. Set aside.

3. Add the cream of tartar to the egg whites and beat on high speed with an electric mixer for about 7 to 9 minutes. Stop when the peaks are stiff but not dry or until the whites no longer slip when bowl is tilted.

4. Stir the egg yolks into the milk-cheese mixture until blended. Gently but thoroughly fold the mixture into the egg whites until no streaks of white remain. Pour the mixture into an ungreased 2-quart soufflé dish or other ceramic dish with sides at least 4 inches high.

5. Bake until soufflé is puffy, delicately browned, and shakes slightly when the oven rack is moved gently back and forth, 30 to 40 minutes. Serve immediately, by cracking open the surface and dishing portions that include both center and crust.

6. While you may store leftovers in the refrigerator for up to 2 days and reheat in the microwave until piping hot, I don't recommend it. Soufflés are best eaten when made. Leftovers will have a dramatically different texture, more dense than airy.

PANCAKES FOR DINNER!

This is basically a tweaked version of my brunch pancake recipe, turning them into crepes for a fun kid-friendly dinner. (My kids call them "pancakes" no matter.) I like to offer a choice of fillings (ideas on page 117) and serve them with Greek yogurt and fruit. If the kids choose to eat them plain, well, at least they are getting ¾ of an egg in each crepe.

The mix can be made up to a day in advance and stored covered in the refrigerator. The cooked crepes are best eaten warm, but cold leftovers can be used as a "wrap" for sandwich fillings—great for lunch boxes! They can also be pureed, with avocado, cooked vegetables, or filling leftovers and frozen for baby to be used within the next month.

Makes 12 medium crepes. Each crepe contains ¾ egg. One and a half crepes, served over the course of a week, provide the weekly egg dose. Two and a half crepes provide about ½ the weekly dairy dose.

9 small eggs
1½ cups whole milk
3 tablespoons butter, melted
¼ teaspoon salt
1¾ cups all-purpose flour

1. In a large bowl, beat the eggs and the milk together. Add the butter and salt. Mix well. Stir in the flour until just incorporated. Batter may be a bit lumpy.

2. Preheat the oven to 175°F.

3. Lightly butter a large griddle or frying pan and place over medium-high heat. Pour or scoop the batter onto the griddle, using approximately ⅓ cup for each crepe.

4. When you see little bubbles forming in the batter, flip and cook until browned. Place on a baking sheet and keep warm in the oven until you are ready to serve.

5. Store leftovers in an airtight container in the refrigerator for 3 to 4 days, or freeze for up to 2 months. Defrost fully at room temperature for an hour or two or overnight in the fridge before using. To reheat, warm them one by one in a microwave or spread out onto baking sheets and place in a 200°F oven for 10 to 15 minutes. Don't stack them because they could stick to one another.

SAVORY FILLING IDEAS:
- Cherry tomatoes, halved, dressed with olive oil, oregano, salt, black pepper, mixed with thinly sliced red onion and feta cheese
- Mushrooms sautéed in butter, with optional minced fresh herbs, such as parsley, chives, thyme, or my favorite, rosemary
- Melted goat cheese or cream cheese, mixed with sautéed spinach (or defrosted frozen spinach), seasoned with chopped garlic, salt, and pepper to taste
- Slices of ripe avocado, cherry tomato, and crumbled bacon
- Crumbled sausage and roasted broccoli florets
- Grated cheddar cheese

PEKING DUCK AND CREPES

Another pancakes-for-dinner recipe inspired by my husband's favorite Chinese dish—Peking duck. I often serve these Chinese-style crepes with stir-fried vegetables and my roasted Easy Duck (page 119), since my children love to gnaw on duck drumsticks, go figure. These crepes can also be wrapped around sausages and called "pigs in a blanket."

Makes 10 crepes. One crepe provides ½ weekly egg dose; serve twice over the week, or mix and match with another recipe to provide the weekly egg dose.

1 Easy Duck (recipe follows)
5 small eggs
½ cup whole milk
⅛ teaspoon salt
1 cup all-purpose flour

1. In a medium bowl, beat together the eggs, milk, salt, and ½ cup water. Stir in the flour until well combined. Batter will be thin with a few lumps.

2. Preheat the oven to 175°F.

3. Heat 1 teaspoon of vegetable oil in an 8- or 9-inch skillet over medium-high heat. When the oil thins and runs easily around the pan, wipe with a paper towel. Making one crepe at a time, ladle in about ¼ cup of the mix; allow the batter to spread to the edges of the pan—you want these to be very thin. When you see little bubbles forming in the batter, it is time to flip the crepe. Place on a baking sheet and keep warm in the oven until you are ready to serve.

4. Store leftover crepes in an airtight container in the refrigerator for up to 3 days, or freeze for up to 2 months. Defrost fully at room temperature for an hour or overnight in the fridge before using. To reheat, warm them one by one in the microwave or spread out onto baking sheets and place in a 200°F oven for 10 to 15 minutes. Don't stack them as they might stick to one another.

EASY DUCK

Rub it, throw it in a hot oven, take it out again. Can it get easier than that?

Makes 3 to 4 servings.

½ tablespoon coarse salt
½ teaspoon freshly ground black pepper
½ teaspoon ground allspice
1 4.5-pound (2 kg) duck
1 orange, halved

1. Preheat the oven to 400°F. Lightly grease a baking sheet with 1 tablespoon of vegetable or olive oil and set aside.

2. In a small bowl, mix together the salt, pepper, and allspice. Randomly prick the skin all over the duck with a fork. Rub the spice mixture over the duck and stuff both orange halves inside. Roast for 20 minutes plus another 20 minutes for every pound (500 g) of the total weight. Let rest for 10 to 20 minutes before carving. If you like, shred some of the meat using two forks.

DESSERT

KID-FRIENDLY EGGNOG

Adult eggnog uses alcohol to help kill possible bacteria, such as salmonella, but a kid-friendly version can be made by slowly cooking the mixture first. I love to use the leftovers to make French toast; simply soak bread in the nog and then pan-fry in butter.

Makes eight ⅔-cup servings.
Two servings provide the weekly egg and dairy doses.

4 small eggs
4 cups whole milk
½ cup sugar
2 teaspoons vanilla extract

1. In a medium bowl, beat together the eggs and milk, then beat in the sugar and vanilla until well incorporated. Pour the mixture into a large heavy-bottomed pot and cook over low heat, stirring constantly, for 5 to 7 minutes, until it thickens slightly and coats the spoon. Do not let the mixture boil.

2. Store leftovers in an airtight container in the refrigerator for up to 1 day. Do not freeze.

MILK CHOCOLATE MOUSSE

This is very popular in our house and it keeps for at least 3 days in the refrigerator, so I can dole it out over several days and get the egg servings in. Many mousse recipes call for raw whipped egg whites, which can be risky for little ones. Here whipped cream lends the necessary volume and silky smooth texture and the eggs have been cooked through in the first step.

The recipe only provides egg-yolk proteins, so you'll have to find another use for the egg whites. Serving the mousse with several Egg-White Meringue Cookies (page 123), made from the leftover egg whites is a fun option.

Makes 8 servings. Each serving contains ½ egg yolk.

4 egg yolks
3 tablespoons sugar
2 cups heavy cream
8 ounces (226 g) milk chocolate
1 teaspoon vanilla extract

1. In a small heavy-bottomed saucepan, whisk together the yolks, 1½ tablespoons of the sugar, and ¾ cup of the cream. Stir over medium-low heat for a few minutes until the mixture thickens slightly and coats the back of the spoon. The aim is to cook the egg yolks to a safe point, but you don't want to boil or curdle. Once thickened, remove the saucepan from the heat.

2. Break the chocolate into chunks and melt gently in a microwave or with a double boiler. Stir into the yolk mixture, then stir in the vanilla.

3. In a medium bowl, whip the remaining 1¼ cups cream and 1½ tablespoons sugar until stiff peaks form. Gently fold the chocolate mixture into the whipped cream. Divide the mousse into 8 ramekins or small bowls and refrigerate for at least 30 minutes.

4. Store leftovers, covered in plastic wrap, in the refrigerator for 3 to 4 days, or freeze for up to 1 month. Defrost in the fridge for 5 to 6 hours before serving. The mousse will have lost some of its volume, but it will still be yummy.

EGG-WHITE MERINGUE COOKIES

Grant calls these "candy"—his highest praise. And with a bit of food coloring you can make them in just about any color you please.

Because this recipe uses only egg whites (see Tip on page 114 for an easy way to separate whites from yolks), you'll need to find another use for the yolks. Pairing these meringues with Milk Chocolate Mousse (page 121) is popular in my house.

This recipe was based on a recipe developed by the spice and flavoring company McCormick & Company. Recipe courtesy of McCormick.

Makes 72 exceptionally light and airy cookies; 18 will provide a week's worth of egg white. If nearly 3 cookies a day seems like too many cookies for a week, no matter how light, mix and match with other egg recipes to reach the weekly quota for egg.

4 egg whites
½ teaspoon cream of tartar
1 cup sugar
1 teaspoon vanilla extract
30 drops food coloring (optional)

1. Preheat the oven to 225°F. Spray two baking sheets with nonstick cooking spray.

2. With an electric mixer, beat the egg whites in a large bowl. When frothy, add the cream of tartar. Continue to beat until you have soft peaks. The egg whites should look like a cloud, and when you pull the mixture up, the bit on the end of the whisk has a droopy point. Add the sugar, vanilla, and if using, the food coloring and beat until stiff peaks form—when you pull the beater up, the little points stay conical.

3. Drop large teaspoonfuls of batter onto the baking sheets about an inch apart. Bake for 45 minutes, until the cookie doesn't wiggle in the middle when the tray is shaken, then turn off the heat. Leave the cookies in the oven for at least another hour, until completely cool. You want these baked all the way through, until they are crispy. They will not brown.

4. Store leftovers in an airtight container at room temperature for 7 to 10 days.

BAKED EGG CUSTARD

This custard smells delicious while baking in the oven; I especially like it with almond extract, but my kids seem to prefer the vanilla version. It is worth making often just to have it perfuming the kitchen!

Makes 2 servings.
Two servings provide the weekly egg and dairy doses.

1 small egg, beaten
⅔ cup whole milk
4 teaspoons sugar
1 teaspoon vanilla or almond extract
Pinch of ground nutmeg or cinnamon (optional)

1. Preheat the oven to 350°F.

2. In a small bowl, whisk or beat together all the ingredients until well mixed. Divide the mixture into two 4-ounce ramekins (or other small ovenproof container). Place the ramekin in a deep oven pan, such as a 10 × 14-inch roasting pan, an 8-inch cake pan, or any other pan with a high rim that is large enough for both ramekins. Fill the pan with water until it reaches about halfway up the sides of the ramekins. Put the pan into the oven and bake for 40 to 50 minutes, until fully set. The mixture should be solid and not run if you tilt the ramekin from side to side.

3. Store leftovers, covered in plastic wrap, in the refrigerator for 3 to 4 days. They do not freeze well.

COCOA CLOUDS

These are actually a variation on chocolate soufflé, but they are so fun to make (and eat), I needed to give them a more playful name. Clara says they taste like "cakey hot chocolate."

Makes 4 servings. Each serving provides ¾ weekly egg dose.

3 small eggs
3.5 ounces (100 g) sweet baking chocolate
5 tablespoons plus 1 teaspoon butter
¼ teaspoon cream of tartar
¼ cup sugar

1. Preheat the oven to 350°F. Separate the eggs (see Tip on page 114), placing the egg whites in a medium bowl and the egg yolks in a small bowl, and set aside. Allow the egg whites to warm to room temperature.

2. Break the chocolate into small pieces and, stirring frequently, melt with the butter in the microwave, a double boiler, or a bowl placed over a pot of gently simmering water. (The water should not touch the bowl or the chocolate could scorch or seize.) Remove from the heat and set aside for a few minutes.

3. Add the cream of tartar to the egg whites and beat together with an electric mixer set at a high speed. Slowly add the sugar while beating. Stop when the peaks are stiff but not dry, or until the whites no longer slip when the bowl is tilted, about 3 to 5 minutes.

4. Stir the egg yolks into the melted chocolate-butter mixture until well incorporated. Gently but thoroughly fold this mixture into the egg whites until no streaks of white remain. Spoon the mixture into 4 quarter-liter (7 fluid-ounce) ramekins, ungreased, filling about two-thirds of the way. If you don't have ramekins for individual servings, the batter can also be baked in a single 1.5- or 2-quart soufflé dish.

5. Bake until the soufflés are puffy, cracked, and no longer have shiny, wet areas, about 20 minutes. If you are using one large soufflé dish, increase the baking time to 40 minutes. They will shake slightly. Classically, you should serve these immediately while they are at peak puffiness, but the ramekins can be quite hot for kids to handle. They are also delicious, and easier to handle, after being allowed to cool for 25 minutes.

6. Store leftovers, covered in plastic wrap, in the refrigerator for up to 3 days, but be aware that they will lose their puff. Serve leftovers cold. Unfortunately, these don't freeze well.

MAKE AHEAD TIP: You can store unbaked soufflés in the refrigerator, covered in plastic wrap, for up to 12 hours and bake before serving. Add 5 minutes to the baking time if baking from chilled.

Recipes for Nut Allergy Prevention

....

We now have plentiful guidelines on peanut allergy prevention, but medical researchers are still working on the exact amounts needed to prevent allergy development of other nuts, including macadamia, walnut, pecan, pine nut, pistachio, almond, and hazelnut. A study investigating these nuts was showing progress when this book went to press. At this time, it is expected, but not yet proven, that early, continual exposure to tree nuts will prevent tree nut allergy, just as evidence suggests that early, continual exposure to other major allergens helps prevent the development of those food allergies.

Introduce nuts under a doctor's supervision or after your baby has been tested for nut allergies, if you have a high-risk baby (i.e., one who has eczema, dry skin, or a family history of allergies or autoimmune disorders). After introduction, continue to feed your baby, toddler, and preschooler tree nuts on a regular, at least twice-weekly, basis.

The chart below delineates the amounts known to protect from peanut allergy over the first five years of life. For tree nuts, we'll have to wait for official recommendations. Estimates of tree nut doses in the below recipes is speculative at best. For now, until we have more data, all we can say is that some exposure to tree nuts is *much* better than no exposure—and likely the more exposure, the better. See "Nut Allergy Prevention Guidelines" in chapter 4 (page 86) for more details.

Peanut	Weekly Amount
Smooth Peanut Butter	3 rounded teaspoons (at least 16 g)
Finely Ground Peanuts	5 level teaspoons (16 g)
Crunchy Peanut Butter (from one year old)	3 rounded teaspoons (at least 16 g)

Weekly doses are the *minimum* a baby or child is advised to eat. It is fine, perhaps even desirable, to surpass the required amounts. From an allergy-prevention perspective, the more a child eats, the better. It is also best if the baby or child is *exposed to each allergen at least twice a week, no matter the amount eaten the first day.* So if your child wolfs down 3 rounded teaspoons of nut butter on Monday, you still need to make sure she eats at least 1½ teaspoons later in the week.

NUTS FOR BABY

 ## SWIRLY PEANUT YOGURT

A peanut butter smoothie! Who says this is only for babies? Add some fruit and sign me up. You could also add a couple teaspoons of homemade tree nut butter (see page 133) to help protect from tree nut allergies simultaneously.

Makes 2 to 4 servings, depending on the size and appetite of your baby. The full recipe provides the weekly peanut and dairy doses, best served over 2 or more days.

3 rounded teaspoons smooth peanut butter
2 teaspoons hot water
½ cup plain full-fat yogurt

1. In a small bowl, thin the peanut butter with the water. Add the peanut butter to the yogurt and mix well. If desired, add in a little pureed fruit or vegetable, such as banana, apple, pear, or sweet potato, for some natural sweetness.

2. Store leftovers in an airtight container in the refrigerator for 3 to 4 days.

PEANUT-TAHINI DIP OR SAUCE

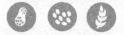

This is a great multitasking recipe. As is, it will protect babies and toddlers from peanut and sesame allergy. Add some soy sauce and a splash of orange juice and you have a yummy dip or sauce for grown-ups, too. You could also add a couple teaspoons of homemade tree nut butter (see page 133) to help protect from tree nut allergies simultaneously.

Makes about 2½ tablespoons of dip or 3 tablespoons of sauce. The full recipe provides the weekly peanut dose and ½ weekly sesame dose. Used as a sauce for pasta, it can help you meet the wheat quota as well (see recipe instructions).

> 3 rounded teaspoons of peanut butter
> 2 to 3 teaspoons hot water (for dip) or 5 to 6 teaspoons (for sauce)
> 1½ teaspoons tahini, well stirred

1. As a dip: In a small bowl, mix the peanut butter and water, then stir in the tahini until well combined. Spread small amounts of the dip onto pieces of soft toast as finger foods for your baby, or serve with rice cakes or cooked and cooled vegetables.

2. As a sauce: In a small bowl, mix the peanut butter and water, then stir in the tahini until well combined. Use as a sauce for rice noodles or pasta. If you cook 1½ ounces (40 g) dried pasta, you can simultaneously meet the weekly wheat requirements.

3. Store leftovers in an airtight container in the refrigerator for 3 days. Can be served warm, cold, or room temperature, as desired.

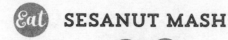

SESANUT MASH

Another multitasking recipe that can be easily turned into a family meal by quadrupling the amounts. Top the puree with charred shrimp skewers and serve with crunchy coleslaw.

Makes about ¾ cup. This recipe provides the weekly sesame and peanut doses, best served over 2 or more days.

3 teaspoons tahini, well stirred
1 small sweet potato, cooked and mashed
3 rounded teaspoons peanut butter

1. In a small bowl, mix together the tahini and mashed cooked sweet potato. Mix in the peanut butter until well combined. Add water, a teaspoon at a time, until the desired consistency is reached.

2. Leftovers can be stored in the refrigerator for up to 48 hours. Alternatively, make it in bulk and freeze in weekly portions for use over the next month.

LUNCH/DINNER/SNACKS

NUT BUTTER PRIMER: BEYOND JIF

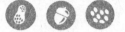

This is my go-to nut allergy prevention weapon. It is easy to find peanut butter, a favorite for many children, and increasingly cashew and almond butter can be found among grocery aisles, particularly in health food stores. But if your aim is to prevent nut allergies—as many nut allergies as possible—in one swift serving, I highly recommend making your own nut butter. The optimum proportion of nuts in this recipe awaits future research, so don't get too bogged down in the exact amounts. The recipe below is simply what I feed my own kids.

If your baby or child already has some nut allergies, take every type of nut that your allergist has deemed safe and blend away. When Clara was still allergic to most nuts, she ate a nut butter made of just her four "safe" nuts every day.

Makes six 12-ounce jars.
Required weekly doses for tree nuts are not currently known. For now, I aim to give my kids at least 15 teaspoons of this a week, to help protect them from peanut, tree nut, and sesame allergies, and I remind myself that for allergy prevention, the more, the better.

5.3 ounces (150 g) walnuts
5.3 ounces (150 g) macadamia nuts
5.3 ounces (150 g) Brazil nuts
5.3 ounces (150 g) cashews
5.3 ounces (150 g) hazelnuts
5.3 ounces (150 g) almonds
3.5 ounces (100 g) pine nuts
3.5 ounces (100 g) pecans

3.5 ounces (100 g) shelled pistachios
12 ounces (340 g) smooth natural peanut butter, well stirred
10.6 ounces (300 g) tahini, well stirred
2 tablespoons walnut or other nut oil (optional)

1. Add all the nuts to a large heavy-duty food processor or high-performance blender. Top with the peanut butter and tahini and blend. If the mixture gets stuck, add the oil. Continue blending until smooth. Spoon into jars, making sure to remove any nut pieces that were not completely blended, as they can be choke hazards for very small children and babies.

2. Store in the refrigerator so that the oils don't separate out, saving you some stirring when you are ready to use the butter. If it does separate, bring the jar to room temperature and just stir the oil back in. Jars can also be stored in the freezer for at least 4 months.

CLEANUP NOTE: I used to gum up the dishwasher after making nut butters. Aside from the fact that it is not good for the dishwasher, you especially want to avoid this if you have another nut allergy in the house at a different stage. The easiest way to get a food processor bowl and blade clean after making a nut butter is to make something else in the container before washing it. If you have a baby, make another puree, something the nut taste will complement, like chicken, potatoes, Asian stir-fry, rice, plain pasta. If your baby is done with puree, grind up fish or turkey and make burgers. Alternatively, grind onions, garlic, fresh ginger, and a bit of sesame oil and orange juice to make an Asian marinade for chicken or pork chops. Washing afterward will be much easier *and* you have a leg up on dinner.

HOMEMADE NUT FLOUR

If your child hates the taste of nuts, the friendliest way to sneak them into his or her diet is through baked goods made with nut flour. Almond flour is easy to find in health food stores, but flour made of other nuts will most likely need to be made at home. (That said, there are some online retailers, such as Nuts.com, that carry an enormous variety of flours, including flours made from nearly all nuts.) Pine nuts are an exception; they turn to "butter" too quickly in the food processor to make a usable flour.

The nuts and food processor should be dry and at room temperature, which will result in a nice fluffy flour. You can use any combination of nuts you want, but grind each one separately in a heavy-duty food processor and then mix together in a large bowl. Nuts have different densities and can differ in how much grinding they need to become flour. The most important point is to avoid overgrinding, or you'll end up with a nut butter instead of nut flour. With softer nuts, such as pecans, you may have to be satisfied with a coarse meal rather than a fine flour, but it can be used as a flour in most recipes and usually adds a nice texture.

If your child already has nut allergies, but there are some nuts that are considered safe, try making a flour of just the safe nuts. Use the flour in the following recipes or substitute half (or more) of the regular flour in your own favorite cookie or cake recipe with nut flour; the result may be slightly more rich and dense but still delicious.

Makes 6 cups. While you need 5 teaspoons of ground peanuts a week to meet the weekly dose, the required weekly doses for tree nuts are not currently known. Judging by the relative protein contents, my best guess is that upward from 6 teaspoons of nut flour could be

required for each tree nut, but research is desperately
needed. For now, just use nut flours liberally and often.

6 cups unsalted, sugar-free plain nuts, such as pistachios,
walnuts, cashews, peanuts, macadamias, hazelnuts, Brazil
nuts, pecans, or almonds—kept separated

1. In a food processor, pulse 2 cups of a single nut variety
about 4 to 8 times, until you have uniform dry flour. Pour
into a large bowl. Add 2 cups of another nut variety to the
food processor. Pulse again until the nuts resemble flour
and add to the bowl. Do the same for one more nut variety,
then stir the nut flours through until combined.

2. Store the flour in an airtight container in the refrigerator
for up to 6 months, or freeze for up to 1 year. I don't recommend using nut flours directly from the freezer, however, as
they tend to clump. Bring to room temperature before using
by leaving on the counter for several hours. Do not attempt
to defrost in the microwave; this will make the flour mushy.

NUT FLOUR CRACKERS

Fun and addictive, this dual-allergy-battling recipe is adapted from a sesame cracker recipe found on the blog of Elana Amsterdam, a paleo cookbook writer. If your kid really likes these (i.e., eats them by the dozen), they will help prevent egg allergy as well.

Makes 96 crackers. Sixteen crackers, served over the course of a week, help protect from sesame and nut allergies and provide ½ weekly egg dose.

3 small eggs
3 cups finely ground Homemade Nut Flour (page 135)
  or store bought
1¼ teaspoons salt
1 cup sesame seeds
2 tablespoons olive oil

1. Preheat the oven to 350°F.

2. In a large bowl, whisk the eggs by hand until lightly frothy, about 1 minute. Add the flour, salt, sesame seeds, and oil and combine well.

3. Cover two 9 × 13-inch baking sheets with parchment paper. Roughly gather the dough into two equal-size balls and put one ball on each sheet. Cover with another sheet of parchment paper and roll out the dough until at least ⅛-inch thick. The dough should cover nearly the whole pan.

4. Remove the top piece of parchment paper and cut the dough with a sharp knife into 2-inch squares. Bake on the middle rack of the oven for 20 to 23 minutes, until golden brown. Allow to cool before peeling off the parchment paper.

5. Store at room temperature in an airtight container for 7 to 10 days.

CRISPY NUT CHICKEN

This is a versatile, freezable recipe that can be made with any variety or mixture of tree nuts and/or peanuts. You can use dry-roasted, honey-roasted, or raw nuts—whatever flavors you think your little ones will like best. Either make Homemade Nut Flour (page 135), or buy nut flour from the store. Almond flour is particularly easy to find. Seasoning ideas include white or black pepper, cumin, sweet smoked paprika, garlic powder, dried herbs, and of course, salt.

The nut flavor is quite mild, but if your child really hates nuts, leave out the crushed nuts (but keep the nut flour) and use five slices of bread for the outermost coating. He will have less nut exposure, but some is better than none. Serve twice in a week or alternate with a different recipe.

Note: Honey may contain bacteria that can't be handled by the digestive system of a child less than one year old, so recipes containing honey should not be served to babies.

Makes 12 mini–chicken fillets.
Two fillets provide about 6 teaspoons of ground
nuts (more if you are using the nuts and not just
the nut flour) and ½ weekly wheat dose.

¾ cup Homemade Nut Flour (page 135) or store bought,
    seasoned to taste
2 small eggs
¾ cup nuts (optional)
3 to 5 slices whole wheat bread (use 5 slices if
    not using nuts)
15 ounces (425 g) skinless, boneless chicken tenders
    or mini-fillets

1. Preheat the oven to 400°F. Grease two baking sheets with a thin coating of olive or vegetable oil, or line them with parchment paper, and set aside.

2. Put the nut flour in a wide, shallow bowl or pie pan. In a second wide, shallow bowl, lightly beat the eggs. In a food processor, combine the nuts and bread into a coarse crumb and place in a third wide, shallow bowl.

3. Working with single pieces, dredge the chicken in the flour, then in the eggs, and lastly in the nut crumbs. Place the coated chicken on the baking sheets, generously spaced from one another. Bake for 20 to 30 minutes (depending on size), flipping halfway, until cooked through and toasty brown. Cut one in half, as a tester, to make sure the chicken is no longer pink inside. Serve with honey mustard, barbecue sauce, or another favorite dip.

4. Store leftovers in an airtight container in the refrigerator for up to 2 days, or freeze for up to 2 months. To reheat, bake from frozen at 300°F for 15 to 20 minutes, flipping halfway through.

NUT BUTTER SATAY

Let the kids help make this easy-peasy, lemon-squeezy recipe. Have them pour in all the ingredients before placing the pan on the stove. Use on noodles, chicken, shrimp, vegetables, or my favorite, fresh pineapple.

Makes about 2 cups. Two rounded tablespoons contain at least 3 teaspoons of nut butter, which, if using peanut butter, provide the weekly peanut dose.

½ cup smooth homemade nut butter (see Nut Butter Primer on page 133) or store-bought nut butter
1 cup whole coconut milk
1 tablespoon soy sauce
3 tablespoons (packed) brown sugar
2 tablespoons freshly squeezed orange, lime, or lemon juice

1. Combine all the ingredients in a small saucepan. Stir over low heat until well combined and the sugar has completely dissolved.

2. Serve warm or cold as a sauce for pasta or as dip for chicken, shrimp, roasted vegetables, or crudités. Store leftovers, covered, in the fridge for 48 hours and serve warm or cold.

NUTTY NOODLES

This Asian-influenced pasta dish can be easily quadrupled to make a family meal for at least two kids and two adults. When I am feeling ambitious, I like to top it with chopped chives, cilantro, and peanuts and serve with a wedge of fresh lime on the side. If I don't have any fish leftovers on hand, a 5-ounce can of light tuna is easily subbed in.

Note: Honey may contain bacteria that can't be handled by the digestive system of a child less than one year old, so recipes containing honey should not be served to babies.

> Makes 2 small servings. Each serving provides the weekly egg, wheat, sesame, peanut, and fish doses and provides protection from tree nut allergy as well.

3 ounces (80 g) or 88 sticks uncooked spaghetti
2 tablespoons tahini, well stirred
2 rounded tablespoons peanut butter
2 tablespoons tree nut butter, such as almond, cashew, or a mix (see Nut Butter Primer on page 133)
1 tablespoon honey
1 tablespoon freshly squeezed orange juice
1 teaspoon soy sauce
1.75 ounces (50 g) cooked fish, such as haddock, cod, tilapia, or salmon
2 small hard-boiled eggs, cooled

1. Boil the spaghetti according to the directions on the package. Drain and set aside.

2. In a small bowl, make the sauce by combining the tahini, peanut butter, tree nut butter, honey, orange juice, and soy sauce with a fork or whisk. Stir well until completely combined. Pour over the pasta and toss, so that the pasta is well coated with the sauce.

3. Break up the fish into small chunks, roughly ½ inch wide. (If your child *really* hates fish, you may want to break it up more so that it isn't visually recognizable.) Stir the fish into the pasta dish. Top with slices of hard-boiled egg. Serve hot or cold.

4. Store leftovers in an airtight container in the refrigerator for up to 3 days. Reheat in a small pot or in the microwave until piping hot.

5. The sauce can also be frozen on its own for use over the next two months. Defrost in the fridge for at least 5 hours. Stir thoroughly before adding to freshly cooked pasta.

DESSERT

CANDY SURPRISE COOKIES

These cookies, adapted from *Sally's Baking Addiction* blog, can be made with your own nut butter or any store-bought variety. They are so tasty that I have to hide them from my kids to make them last! The nut taste in the cookie is mild, but if your child truly hates anything with a nutty flavor, hiding chocolate candy in the middle masks the nut taste completely.

Makes 20 cookies.

To fight both peanut and tree nut allergy, use a mixed-nut butter that combines nuts, such as the one on page 133. If you instead opt to use just peanut butter, 1½ cookies over the course of a week will more than satisfy the peanut dose. With a mixed-nut butter, where the doses for tree nuts are currently unknown, I'd just aim for 1 or 2 a day, especially if this is the only tree nut exposure your child is getting.

    8 tablespoons (1 stick) salted butter, softened to room
        temperature
    ½ cup (packed) light brown sugar
    1 medium egg
    ¾ cup smooth homemade nut butter (see Nut Butter Primer
        on page 133) or store-bought nut butter
    1 teaspoon vanilla extract
    ½ teaspoon baking soda
    1¼ cups all-purpose flour
    20 chocolate candies, such as Hershey's Kisses or
        Rolo chocolate-covered caramels

1. Cream the butter and sugar together with a mixer. Add the egg, nut butter, and vanilla and mix well. Stir in baking soda and flour until well incorporated. Refrigerate for at least 30 minutes, or if not baking right away, freeze the batter for up to 3 months.

2. Preheat the oven to 350°F. Lightly grease two baking sheets with butter and set aside.

3. For each cookie, roll a small ball (1½ to 2 tablespoons) of batter. Cut the ball in half and press the candy in on one side. Top with the other half of the ball and place on the prepared baking sheets. Bake for 10 minutes. Once cooled, hide!

4. If your family has more discipline than mine and can manage not to eat the whole batch in one day, store leftovers in an airtight container for 7 to 10 days at room temperature, or freeze for up to 2 months. Defrost at room temperature for at least 1 hour before serving.

NUT FLOUR SHORTBREAD

These cookies couldn't be easier to make. I prepare them with almond flour, and Clara, who hates almonds, loves them. Any nut flour will work; just make sure it is ground to at least the consistency of a fine cornmeal (not to be confused with cornstarch); don't overgrind, however, or you will get nut butter.

You can make several batches of dough and leave unbaked portions in the freezer until you're ready to use. Then just slice and bake as needed (defrosting not required).

For variation, or if your kid doesn't like chocolate, you can sub in additional nut flour for the cocoa. For adults, or more adventurous children, ⅓ cup dried fruit or whole nuts can be added, but for allergy-fighting purposes, I'd leave lumpy additions out as I find younger children are more likely to enjoy baked goods that are one consistent texture.

Makes 10 cookies.
Each cookie contains about 4 teaspoons of ground nut flour. If using a peanut flour, your child needs to eat at least 1¼ of these each week. If you are using a mixed-nut flour (recommended), because the doses for tree nuts are currently unknown, I'd just aim for one or two cookies a day, especially if this is the only tree nut exposure your child is getting.

3 tablespoons butter, melted
½ teaspoon vanilla extract
¾ cup plus 2 tablespoons finely ground
    Homemade Nut Flour (page 135) or store bought
2 tablespoons cocoa powder
3 tablespoons confectioners' sugar
⅛ teaspoon salt
⅛ teaspoon ground cinnamon (optional)

1. In a large bowl, combine the butter and vanilla. In a medium bowl, combine the flour, cocoa powder, sugar, salt, and if using, cinnamon, and then mix the dry ingredients into the butter mixture. There's no need to get out the mixer for this—a fork works fine. Stir until the dough is stiff and a bit like Play-Doh. Make a log, about 7½ inches long and 2 inches in diameter, and wrap in plastic wrap. Place in the freezer for at least 30 minutes, until the dough is hard. Or freeze for up to 2 months before continuing on as described below.

2. Preheat the oven to 350°F.

3. Prepare a baking sheet with parchment paper or grease it lightly. Slice the chilled unwrapped log into ¾-inch rounds and place flat on the sheet about 1 inch apart; they tend not to spread. Bake for 14 minutes. Allow to cool *on the sheet* for at least 10 minutes before removing or they will crumble. Once they are cool, they are hardy—and delicious.

4. Store leftovers in an airtight container for 7 to 10 days at room temperature, or freeze for up to 2 months. Defrost at room temperature for at least 1 hour before serving.

NUT FLOUR CHOCOLATE TORTE

This rich, dense cake is pure and simple—no frosting required or even desired. I have yet to make this last in our house for more than a day, because everyone begs for seconds!

Makes 16 small slices. Each slice has 3 teaspoons nut flour. Serve 2 slices over 2 days to provide the weekly peanut dose, if using only ground peanut flour. If using a tree nut flour or mixed-nut flour (recommended), this recipe will help protect against tree nut allergy as well. Each slice also provides ¼ egg dose.

1 cup semisweet chocolate chips
8 tablespoons (1 stick) butter, plus more for greasing
4 small eggs
¼ teaspoon cream of tartar
¾ cup sugar
1 teaspoon vanilla extract
¼ teaspoon salt
1 cup finely ground Homemade Nut Flour (page 135)
    or store bought

1. Preheat the oven to 350°F. Lightly grease a 9-inch cake pan with butter and set aside.

2. Place the chocolate chips in a medium microwave-safe bowl. Slice the butter and add to the chocolate. Microwave on low, checking and stirring frequently until chocolate is completely melted. (You could also do this using a double boiler, but I find the microwave technique more forgiving if I get interrupted by a small child.)

3. Separate the eggs (see Tip on page 114), putting the yolks and whites in two different large bowls. Add the cream of tartar to the egg whites and whip until stiff peaks form, that is, until you can raise the beater and see little points that instead of drooping stay conical. Add the sugar, vanilla, and salt to the egg yolks and mix well. Stir the nut flour and melted chocolate into the yolk mixture. Slowly fold in your cloud of whipped egg whites, stirring until the mixture is one uniform color. Do not overstir. Transfer batter to the prepared cake pan.

4. Bake for 35 minutes, or until set and slightly cracked in the middle. Cool completely on a wire rack before slicing, for 2 to 3 hours. Slice with a sharp knife; to get pretty, neat slices, wipe the knife clean after each cut. Serve with whipped cream.

5. Store leftovers in an airtight container in the refrigerator for 3 to 4 days, or freeze for 1 month. Defrost overnight in the fridge before serving.

Recipes for Sesame Allergy Prevention

Sesame	Weekly Amount
Tahini	3 teaspoons (15 g)
Hummus*	About 8 rounded tablespoons (120 g)
Sesame Seeds	About 8 heaped teaspoons (22 g)

Make sure the hummus ingredient list includes tahini or sesame.

Weekly doses are the *minimum* a baby or child is currently advised to eat. It is fine, perhaps even desirable, to surpass the required amounts. It is also best if the baby or child is *exposed to each allergen at least twice a week, no matter the amount eaten the first day.* So if your child wolfs down 3 teaspoons of tahini on Monday, you still need to make sure she eats at least 1½ teaspoons later in the week.

SESAME FOR BABY

 # OPEN SESAME SWEET POTATO PUREE

This is among the very small number of baby foods I'd actually want to eat myself. I have, in fact, served it to adults, alongside grilled chicken and shrimp.

Makes about 3 cups. Half the recipe provides the weekly sesame dose and, if the milk is used, the weekly dairy dose, too. It is best served over 2 or more days.

2 small sweet potatoes (about 10 ounces total), scrubbed and peeled
6 teaspoons tahini, well stirred
1⅓ cups whole milk or water

1. Preheat the oven to 400°F. Lightly grease a baking sheet with 1 teaspoon olive oil and set aside.

2. Chop the sweet potatoes into rough 1-inch cubes and place on the baking sheet. Roast in the oven until very tender, about 30 minutes.

3. In a medium bowl, mash the potatoes with a fork or run through the food processor. Stir or blend in the tahini, then the milk, mixing until well combined.

4. Store half in an airtight container in the refrigerator for use over the week. Freeze the other half for up to 2 months.

HUMMUS-TAHINI DIP

Traditionally, hummus already contains some sesame in the form of tahini, but I've noticed some brands leave it out. Check the ingredient list of store-bought hummus for tahini or sesame (or make your own; see Hummus on page 158) to ensure this recipe gives an adequate dose of sesame. Toddlers, big kids, and adults may like this dip, too.

Makes 5 tablespoons of dip, or about 2 servings.
This recipe provides the weekly sesame dose,
best served over 2 or more days.

1½ teaspoons tahini, well stirred
1½ teaspoons hot water
4 tablespoons Hummus (page 158) or store bought

1. In a small bowl, thin the tahini with the water. Then mix in the hummus. Either spoon-feed to baby, or use as a dip with thin slices of well-cooked and cooled vegetables such as carrots, green beans, bell peppers, or small pieces of pita bread.

2. Store leftovers in an airtight container in your refrigerator for up to 4 days. If you are fine with losing a bit of the fluffy quality of the hummus (I barely notice it), the dip will keep in your freezer for up to 2 months. Defrost overnight in the fridge before serving.

BUTTERNUT SQUASH HUMMUS

This freezer-friendly recipe takes the classic hummus recipe of ground chickpeas and tahini and gives it a baby-friendly spin. Replacing the chickpeas with roasted butternut squash gives the puree some natural sweetness to offset the slight bitterness of the tahini.

Makes about 2 cups. Half of this recipe provides the weekly sesame dose, best served over 2 or more days.

1 2-pound butternut squash
2 garlic cloves, each sliced into 3 pieces
Sprinkle of minced fresh rosemary or dried (optional)
2 teaspoons olive oil
6 teaspoons tahini, well stirred

1. Preheat the oven to 400°F. Line a baking sheet with aluminum foil and set aside.

2. Peel the butternut squash with a carrot peeler. Separate the bulbous part of the squash from the long stem end. Cut the bulbous part in half and scoop out the seeds, along with their stringy bits, with a spoon. Discard the seeds. Remove the stem from the other half.

3. Roughly chop the prepared squash into 1-inch cubes. You should have about 3 cups. Put the squash, garlic, and rosemary in a medium bowl, drizzle with oil, and toss to coat. Place the squash mixture onto the prepared baking sheet and roast in the oven for 20 to 25 minutes, until soft. Remove from the oven and let cool.

4. After the squash has cooled, remove the garlic pieces and then blend the rest with 2 tablespoons water to make a pureed texture. Thoroughly mix in the tahini.

5. Serve on its own or use as a dip with thin slices of soft-cooked and cooled vegetables like carrots, green beans, and bell peppers or even with small pieces of pita bread.

6. Store leftovers in the refrigerator for 3 to 4 days, or freeze for up to 2 months. Defrost in the fridge for at least 5 hours before serving.

TIP: If your child is already comfortable eating mashed or lumpy textures, you will not need to blend the butternut squash smooth.

LUNCH/DINNER/SNACKS

SAVORY FALAFEL "COOKIES"

Okay, I like to think of these as "cookies" because I cut them with woodland-creature cookie cutters, "frost" them with hummus, and decorate with seeds and currants. But, if I am honest, my kids disagree. These are tasty, but not sweet, and according to Clara and Grady, a cookie is not a cookie if it isn't sweet. Fair enough. If pressed, I just call them lunch instead. And a fun one at that.

Makes twelve ½-inch-thick "cookies." The entire recipe provides the weekly sesame dose. "Frosting" the shapes with hummus will help you meet the quota quicker. These treats can be pan-fried or baked, depending on your preference.

1½ cups chickpea flour
1 teaspoon ground cumin
½ teaspoon salt
½ teaspoon garlic powder
¼ teaspoon white pepper
8 heaped teaspoons sesame seeds
1¼ cups boiling water
2 tablespoons olive oil
⅓ cup Hummus (page 158) or Rainbow Hummus
    (page 159) or store-bought or plain Greek yogurt
    (optional)
1 teaspoon sesame seeds, for decorating (optional)

1. Preheat the oven to 350°F.

2. In a medium bowl, combine the flour, cumin, salt, garlic powder, pepper, and sesame seeds. Stir in the boiling water, then cool for 15 minutes.

3. Mold the mixture into patties, balls, or fingers, or use cookie cutters to make a selection of fun shapes. Stick shapes are great for older babies and young toddlers. Preschoolers appreciate more complicated shapes and characters.

4. Heat the oil in a large skillet or sauté pan. Pan-fry the cookies for 2 minutes on each side. Alternatively, lightly coat a baking sheet with the oil and place the cookies on top about 1 inch apart from one another. Bake for 20 minutes, or until toasty brown.

5. Allow the cookies to cool for 10 to 15 minutes. Let the kids "frost" them at the table with the hummus and sprinkle the top with more sesame seeds.

6. Store unfrosted cookies in an airtight container in the refrigerator for up to 3 days, or freeze for up to 2 months. Defrost at room temperature for at least 2 hours before serving.

SESAME FISH FINGERS

This freezable recipe is a variation on the previous recipe, allowing you to battle both sesame and fish allergies in one go. Serve with Tahini-Honey Dip (page 160) to reach the sesame quota, or pair with other sesame recipes such as Tahini Brownies (page 161) for dessert.

Makes 16 fish sticks, or about 8 toddler-size servings.
Two servings, or ¼ recipe, provide
¼ sesame dose and 4 fish doses.

1½ cups chickpea flour
1 teaspoon ground cumin
½ teaspoon salt
½ teaspoon garlic powder
¼ teaspoon freshly ground black pepper or
   white pepper
8 heaped teaspoons sesame seeds
4 haddock fillets (14 ounces, or 400 g, total),
   cut into 4 strips each
4 tablespoons olive oil

1. In a large bowl, combine the flour, cumin, salt, garlic powder, pepper, and sesame seeds. Dredge the fish strips in the mixture, making sure the fish is coated on all sides. If using fresh haddock, you can freeze the coated fish at this step for up to 6 months. Defrost overnight in the fridge before continuing with below.

2. Working in two batches, heat half the oil in a skillet or sauté pan and then pan-fry half of the coated fish strips for 3 to 4 minutes on each side, until golden brown and fish is cooked through. To see if the fish is ready, break a tester in half and check that the flesh is opaque and firm. Repeat with the second batch.

3. Alternatively, lightly coat two baking sheets with the oil and divide the coated fish strips between both pans, placing them about 2 inches apart from one another. Bake at 350°F for 20 minutes, flipping halfway through, until the fish sticks are a toasty brown.

4. Store leftovers in an airtight container in the refrigerator for up to 3 days. Reheat in a 300°F oven for 15 minutes, flipping halfway through.

HUMMUS

Making hummus from scratch takes only a few minutes. (If you've heard you have to fiddle around taking the thin skins off the chickpeas, you don't.) And it keeps well in the freezer. Freezing changes the consistency ever so slightly, but it is still very tasty. Freeze plain hummus in weekly portions for defrosting later in the month.

**Makes about 4 cups. Four tablespoons
provide the weekly sesame dose.**

⅔ cup freshly squeezed lemon juice (from about 4 lemons)
     or, in a pinch, orange juice from a carton
1 cup tahini, well stirred
3 cups jarred or canned chickpeas, rinsed
4 tablespoons olive oil
Salt to taste

1. In a blender or food processor, add all the ingredients and blend until smooth.

2. Store leftovers in an airtight container in the refrigerator for up to 5 days, or freeze for 2 months.

STORAGE TIP: Freeze plain hummus in weekly portions in small, freezer-safe storage bags. Press out the additional air so that they'll take up less room in your freezer.

RAINBOW HUMMUS

I love adding peppers or berries (or even just some food coloring) to make brightly colored hummus. Getting creative with the colors can be a fun way to make your child feel in control of what he eats when you ask him, "What color hummus should we make this week?"

Makes about 2 cups. Eight tablespoons of the recipe is needed to meet the weekly sesame quota. If using food coloring alone, and leaving the peppers or berries out, 4 tablespoons should suffice. Serve at least twice over the week.

2 roasted bell peppers (see Tip below) or
1½ cups fresh berries, in your favorite colors
1 cup Hummus (page 158)

1. Puree the peppers or berries with the hummus in a food processor until smooth. If the colors aren't vibrant enough for your clan, or they don't like berries and peppers, try a few drops of food coloring.

2. Store leftovers in an airtight container in the refrigerator for 3 days, or freeze for up to 2 months. Defrost for at least 5 hours before serving.

TIP: To roast peppers preheat the oven to 475°F. Rinse whole peppers and poke a hole in each one to let steam escape. Place on an oiled baking sheet and roast for at least 30 minutes, flipping once, until each pepper is starting to collapse. It is fine, even desirable, if the skin chars in places. Let cool. Discard the stems, seeds, and released water before pureeing with the hummus.

TAHINI-HONEY DIP

Serve this dip with crudités and breadsticks, spread on toast, or serve alongside fish fingers or chicken tenders. It can also be used to make cookie sandwiches by spreading 2 teaspoons between graham crackers or other thin cookies.

Note: Honey may contain bacteria that can't be handled by the digestive system of a child less than one year old, so recipes containing honey should not be served to babies.

Makes six 1-tablespoon servings. Your child needs to eat at least 1½ tablespoons, spread over 2 servings, to satisfy the weekly sesame dose.

¼ cup tahini, well stirred
1 tablespoon honey
1 tablespoon freshly squeezed orange juice

1. In a small bowl, mix together all the ingredients by hand, using a fork or whisk.

2. Store leftovers in an airtight container in the refrigerator for up to 3 days. Or make in bulk and freeze in ⅓-cup portions for up to 2 months. Defrost overnight in the fridge and stir well before serving.

DESSERT

TAHINI BROWNIES

I crave these brownies more than any other dessert. They're so delicious and easy to make, and nobody will even guess sesame is a major ingredient. If you are working on desensitizing an egg allergy or simply don't have eggs in the house, the eggs can be omitted, but the result will be more crumbly. If you leave out the eggs, be especially careful not to overbake; start checking the brownies after 20 minutes of baking.

**Makes 24 brownies. Your child needs to eat
at least 1½ brownies, best served over 2 days,
to receive the weekly sesame dose.**

Cocoa powder, for the baking pan
10.6 ounces (300 g) high-quality dark chocolate, such as
    Green & Black's 70 or 85 percent dark chocolate
1 cup freshly squeezed orange juice or whole milk
1 cup tahini, well stirred
½ teaspoon vanilla extract
2 eggs, beaten (optional)
1 cup all-purpose flour
¾ teaspoon baking powder
½ teaspoon salt
1 cup confectioners' sugar

1. Preheat the oven to 350°F. Grease a 9 × 13-inch baking pan with butter and dust with cocoa powder. Set aside.

2. Break the chocolate into small chunks in a small bowl and set aside. Pour ½ cup of the juice into a small saucepan.

Heat gently, then add the chocolate. Melt the chocolate into the liquid over low heat, stirring constantly. Be careful not to overheat or the chocolate will seize. Think "low and slow."

3. In a large bowl, thin the tahini with the remaining ½ cup juice. Add the melted chocolate, vanilla, and if using, the eggs and mix well. In a medium bowl, stir together the flour, baking powder, salt, and sugar until well combined. Add the dry ingredients to the tahini-chocolate mixture and stir well to make a smooth batter. Spread this batter into the prepared pan. Bake for 25 minutes, or until a toothpick inserted into the middle comes out clean.

4. Allow to cool for at least 1 hour. Cut into 24 squares and serve.

5. Store leftovers in an airtight container at room temperature for 2 to 3 days. Alternatively, freeze portions for up to 2 months. Defrost at room temperature for 2 hours before serving.

TAHINI BLONDIES

The tahini gives these bar cookies a mysterious complexity, the origin of which will go unguessable by even the most sesame adverse. I love these. And so do my kids.

Makes 12 blondies. Two blondies, served over the course of a week, provide the weekly sesame dose. Three blondies provide ½ the weekly egg dose.

5 tablespoons plus 1 teaspoon butter, melted
6 tablespoons tahini, well stirred
¾ cup (packed) light brown sugar
2 eggs, beaten
1 teaspoon vanilla extract
1 teaspoon salt
1 cup all-purpose flour
¾ cup chocolate chips (optional)

1. Preheat the oven to 350°F. Grease an 8-inch square deep baking pan or casserole dish with butter.

2. Using a hand mixer, in a large bowl, combine the butter, tahini, and sugar, mixing at a medium speed until smooth, about 1 minute. Then add the eggs, vanilla, and salt and mix until you have a runny, uniform consistency, about 1 minute. Stir in the flour until just combined and, if using, half of the chocolate chips. Spread the batter into the pan. Sprinkle the remaining chocolate chips on top. Bake for 35 to 40 minutes, until a toothpick inserted into the middle comes out clean. Once cool, cut into 12 bars.

3. Store leftovers in an airtight container at room temperature for 2 to 3 days, or freeze portions for up to 2 months. Defrost at room temperature for 2 hours before serving.

TIP: My babies have all hated the sound of a mixer. You can combine the above by hand, using a handheld whisk, if you are willing to give it a minute or two of elbow grease.

Recipes for Dairy Allergy Prevention

Dairy Product	Weekly Amount
Plain Yogurt*	2 1.5-ounce (40g) containers
Plain Thick-Style Greek Yogurt†	4 tablespoons (¼ cup); about 2 ounces (60 g)
Full-Fat Cottage Cheese	2 tablespoons (⅛ cup); about 1 ounce (30 g)
Whole Milk	⅔ cup (150 ml)
Mini Round Cheeses	2 round cheeses, together weighing 1.5 ounces (40 g)
Hard Cheeses	2 cubes, together weighing 0.5 ounce (16 g)
Processed Cheese Slices	About ⅔ a standard slice, weighing 0.5 ounce (16 g)
Mozzarella Ball	0.85 ounce (24 g)

*If using a multiserving container of plain yogurt, try for 7 or 8 large spoonfuls, or about a half cup, a week.

†Strained, thick-style Greek yogurt should have about 9 grams of protein per 100 grams. Runnier nonstrained varieties have half that amount and are comparable to regular yogurts. If using a multiserving container of nonstrained Greek yogurt, with around 4.5 grams of protein per 100 grams, aim for 7 or 8 large spoonfuls a week.

Weekly doses are the *minimum* a baby or child is currently advised to eat. It is fine, perhaps even desirable, to surpass the required amounts. It is also best if the baby or child is *exposed to each allergen at least twice a week, no matter the amount eaten the first day.* So if your child wolfs down 2 Babybels on Monday, you still need to make sure she eats at least 1 Babybel (or ½ dose from a different dairy category) later in the week.

Please note that to be nutritionally adequate, all dairy products should be full fat for children under two years old.

DAIRY FOR BABY

Introducing baby to dairy is pretty easily accomplished with a runny yogurt. We almost always have strained Greek yogurt in our fridge, but I have found this to be too thick for tiny infants. My babies have found regular, nonstrained yogurt a treat. Just make sure it is unsweetened ("plain" or "natural") and full fat or "whole."

 SUNRISE YOGURT

This recipe, for some reason, makes me picture little infant body builders, slurping down their egg protein shake before hitting the baby gym.

Makes about ¾ cup. The full recipe provides the weekly egg and dairy doses, best served over 2 or more days.

1 small hard-boiled egg
1 to 2 tablespoons water
½ cup plain full-fat yogurt

1. Using a food processor, blender, or immersion blender, puree the egg and water until it resembles a smooth paste. Mix in the yogurt and serve. If your baby is on lumpier mashed textures, try fork-mashing the hard-boiled egg with yogurt instead.

2. Store leftovers in an airtight container in the refrigerator for up to 2 days, or freeze for up to 1 month.

BASIC CHEESE SAUCE

This versatile, and freezable, sauce can be used as a yummy allergy-fighting liquid, helping you smooth out purees of other foods (including allergens). It is also just plain good. Toddlers, preschoolers, and even adults will happily eat it when poured over pasta (think mac and cheese) or lightly steamed broccoli.

Makes about 1½ cups, or about 6 servings.
This recipe provides 3 weekly dairy doses.

2 tablespoons butter or oil
2 teaspoons all-purpose flour
⅔ cup whole milk
4 heaping tablespoons grated cheddar cheese

1. Melt the butter in a small sauté pan over low heat, then thoroughly stir in the flour, about 1 minute. Gradually add in the milk, stirring constantly, until the sauce visibly thickens, enough to coat the back of a spoon. This should take about 3 minutes. Remove from the heat. Add the cheese, a little at a time, stirring until it is melted into the sauce.

2. Divide equally into three portions. Store one portion in an airtight container in the refrigerator to use over the next week, and freeze the other two portions for up to 3 months.

3. Serve with cooked vegetables or a ½ pasta or fish dose, pureed for a baby to the desired consistency.

LUNCH/DINNER/SNACK

LABNEH DIP

It sounds exotic, and it is based on a traditional Lebanese food. But at its heart, this is simply yogurt, doubly strained so the proteins are that much more compact, making it a tasty and efficient way to prevent dairy allergy. The recipe makes quite a bit of dip—because I think the adults in the house might want to eat it, too.

Note: Honey may contain bacteria that can't be handled by the digestive system of a child less than one year old, so recipes containing honey should not be served to babies.

Makes 2 cups. Three tablespoons, served over the course of a week, help prevent dairy allergy.

3 cups plain full-fat thick-style Greek yogurt
1 tablespoon freshly squeezed orange or lemon juice
1 tablespoon honey
Salt

1. Line a sieve with cheesecloth. Place the sieve over a medium bowl. Add the yogurt to the sieve and gather the cloth on top to cover the yogurt. Leave in your refrigerator for at least 12 hours, letting the water from the yogurt drain into the bowl.

2. When the yogurt has reduced by a third and is nearly the consistency of whipped cream cheese, scrape it from the cloth into a fresh bowl and stir in the juice and honey. Season with salt to taste. Serve with toasted pita chips and crudités.

3. Store leftovers in an airtight container in the refrigerator for up to 5 days, or freeze up to 2 months. Defrost overnight in the fridge and stir well before serving. Do keep in mind, however, freezing will change the consistency slightly, and some kids who love the freshly made dip may reject the defrosted version.

CHEESY TREATS

Not sure how to classify these . . . They aren't sweet, but they are otherwise a cookie. My daughter calls them grilled cheese cookies, but everyone else just says, "More please!"

I like them as dessert, topped with a bit of jam or honey, but the kids prefer them as a snack. Inspiration for this recipe was taken from Amy Johnson's blog site *She Wears Many Hats*.

Note: Honey may contain bacteria that can't be handled by the digestive system of a child less than one year old, so recipes containing honey should not be served to babies.

Makes 28 cookies. Two cookies provide the
weekly dairy dose, best served over 2 days.

2 cups grated cheddar cheese
2 cups all-purpose flour
4 cups Rice Krispies cereal
1½ sticks butter, melted
2 eggs, beaten

1. Preheat the oven to 325°F. Combine all the ingredients in a large bowl. Form the dough into 28 firm balls, the size of golf balls. Distribute over two greased baking sheets and press flat.

2. Bake for 25 minutes, or until lightly browned. Allow to cool for at least 20 minutes before serving.

3. Store leftovers in an airtight container at room temperature for up to 6 days, or freeze for up to 3 months. Defrost at room temperature for several hours before serving.

VARIATION: Add 1 teaspoon of dried herbs, such as oregano, basil, or sage, to half the batter to offer a selection of flavors.

EGGY CHEESE SOLDIERS

A word of caution: Don't call these soldiers if you don't allow your children to play with food. Otherwise, they will surely be marching up and down the table, or at least around their plates, before they march right into a child's mouth.

**Makes 4 "soldiers," or 1 to 2 servings
depending on the age of the child. The full recipe
provides the weekly dairy, wheat, and egg doses.**

1 egg, beaten
1 thick slice plain whole grain bread
1 tablespoon vegetable oil or butter
2 tablespoons grated cheddar or other hard mild cheese

1. Pour the egg in a wide, shallow bowl or pie pan, then soak the bread in it, flipping once, until the bread is completely saturated and nearly all the liquid is gone. Heat the oil in a large skillet over medium heat and fry the bread until the egg coating is well cooked, about 2 minutes on each side. Sprinkle on the cheese and allow to melt. Cut lengthwise into four little toast "soldiers."

2. Store leftovers in an airtight container in the refrigerator for use over the next 3 days. Warm up thoroughly, in a microwave or toaster oven, before serving leftovers. Unfortunately, these don't freeze well.

FAUX-FRIED CHEESE FINGERS

There is no substitute for halloumi cheese, I am afraid. We call it squeaky cheese in our house due to the sound it makes when chewed. It handles heat differently than other cheeses, making these cheese fingers easy-peasy to make in an oven rather than a deep fryer. If you have trouble finding halloumi cheese in your usual grocery store, try Trader Joe's, Whole Foods, or Amazon.com.

Makes 18 cheese fingers.
One stick provides the weekly dairy dose (16 g
cheese) and ¼ wheat dose or, if using a nut flour
instead, some protection from tree nut allergy.

10.6 ounces (300 g) halloumi cheese (2 standard packages)
1 cup finely ground Homemade Nut Flour (page 135) or dried
   bread crumbs (to make them yourself, see my Bread
   Crumb Primer on page 186)
¼ teaspoon freshly ground black pepper
½ teaspoon dried oregano
½ teaspoon dried thyme

1. Preheat the oven to 400°F. Lightly grease a 13 × 9-inch baking sheet with oil or butter and set aside.

2. Cut the halloumi into sticks, 3 inches long, ½ inch wide, and ½ inch deep. Put the flour in a wide, shallow bowl or pie pan and stir in the pepper, oregano, and thyme. Dredge each halloumi stick in the flour and place on the prepared baking sheet. Bake for at least 30 minutes, flipping halfway, until crispy.

3. Store leftovers in an airtight container in the refrigerator for up to 3 days, reheating in the toaster oven or a 200°F oven for 5 to 8 minutes. Alternatively, freeze the dredged, unbaked halloumi for up to 3 months. Defrost overnight in the fridge and then reheat as described above before serving.

YOGURT MASHED POTATOES

This creamy, slightly tangy mash goes well with just about any roasted or grilled meat. No one will guess there is yogurt in them and your child needs to eat only ½ cup, twice a week, to meet the dairy requirement. If you can't find russet potatoes, Yukon Gold will also work well.

Makes about 4 kid-size ½-cup servings.
Two servings provide the weekly dairy dose.

1 pound Idaho russet potatoes, scrubbed, peeled, and
    halved or, if large, quartered
1 tablespoon butter
½ cup plain full-fat thick-style Greek yogurt
Garlic powder
Freshly ground black pepper

1. In a 6- or 7-quart heavy-bottomed pot, put the potatoes in enough water to cover completely and bring to a boil. Reduce to a simmer and cook for 10 to 15 minutes, until tender. Drain the potatoes in a colander, then place in a large bowl. Add the butter and mash. (If you use a mixer to mash, be careful not to get overzealous or you'll get glue; a few lumps are fine.) Stir in yogurt, season to taste with garlic powder and black pepper, and serve.

2. Store leftovers in an airtight container in the refrigerator for up to 2 days, or freeze individual servings in freezer-safe plastic bags for up to 2 months. You can reheat these from frozen or after thawing overnight in the fridge. Either way, reheat on the stove or in the microwave, warming over low heat and stirring occasionally, until the mash is piping hot.

MAPLE YOGURT MARINATED CHICKEN

My son loves chicken skin, but my daughter loathes it. This recipe can be made with skin on or removed before marinating. Sometimes I'll do half with and half without, allowing a choice at the dinner table. Only about 1 tablespoon yogurt remains on each piece of chicken. Serve liberally with Yogurt-Fruit Chutney (page 174) or serve alongside Yogurt Biscuits (page 176) to meet the weekly dairy quota.

Makes 12 drumsticks, or about 6 servings. One drumstick provides about ⅛ weekly dairy dose.

2½ cups plain full-fat yogurt
2 tablespoons pure maple syrup
½ teaspoon salt
¼ teaspoon smoked paprika
¼ teaspoon garlic powder
12 chicken drumsticks

1. In a large bowl or storage container, combine the yogurt, syrup, salt, paprika, and garlic powder, then add the drumsticks. Cover and refrigerate. Allow the chicken to marinate in the yogurt mixture for at least 2 hours and up to 24 hours.

2. Preheat the oven to 450°F.

3. Lightly coat a roasting pan with olive oil. Place the chicken in the prepared pan, and top with a few spoonfuls of marinade. Roast for 35 to 40 minutes, until the marinade has set and the chicken has cooked through. To check if the chicken is done, prick 1 drumstick with a knife to the bone; if the juices run clear, dinner is ready.

4. Store leftovers in an airtight container in the refrigerator for up to 4 days. Reheat in a microwave for a minute or so, or wrap in foil and reheat in 250°F oven for 15 to 20 minutes.

YOGURT-FRUIT CHUTNEY

Pretty much any fruit will work in this kid-friendly, allergy-fighting version of the Indian staple. Ripe pears or bananas are particularly popular in my house. In a pinch, a couple tablespoons of jam could replace the fruit. This is delicious on chicken or as a dip alongside crudités, toasted pita bread, or papadum.

Note: Honey may contain bacteria that can't be handled by the digestive system of a child less than one year old, so recipes containing honey should not be served to babies.

Makes two 3½-tablespoon servings. The full recipe provides the weekly dairy dose, best served over 2 or more days.

¼ cup plain full-fat thick-style Greek yogurt
⅛ cup minced fresh fruit
1 tablespoon ginger curd or honey
⅛ teaspoon garlic salt
Freshly ground black pepper to taste

1. In a small bowl, stir together all the ingredients until well mixed, then serve.

2. Store leftovers in an airtight container in the refrigerator for up to 2 days, mixing well before serving again.

HONEY-MUSTARD YOGURT DIP

This recipe couldn't be simpler and it's a hit served with crudités, sesame breadsticks, and Couscous-Coated Chicken (page 189) or spread on fish.

Note: Honey may contain bacteria that can't be handled by the digestive system of a child less than one year old, so recipes containing honey should not be served to babies.

Makes six 2-tablespoon servings. Half the recipe provides the weekly dairy dose, best served over 2 or more days.

½ cup plain full-fat thick-style Greek yogurt
2 tablespoons honey
2 tablespoons Dijon or other mild mustard

1. In a small bowl, stir together all the ingredients until well mixed, then serve.

2. Store leftovers in an airtight container in the refrigerator for up to 5 days.

YOGURT BISCUITS

I adapted a recipe found on the Stonyfield website to create this dairy-allergy-fighting side dish. Simple, fluffy comfort food, these biscuits make an easy dinner side or a quick morning treat served with butter and jam.

Makes 16 small biscuits.
Half the recipe, served over the course of a
week, provides the weekly dairy dose.

2 cups flour
¼ teaspoon baking soda
3 teaspoons baking powder
1 teaspoon salt
4 tablespoons (½ stick) butter, melted
1 cup plain full-fat yogurt

1. Preheat the oven to 375°F. Lightly grease two baking sheets with butter and set aside.

2. In a large bowl, combine the flour, baking soda, baking powder, and salt. In a small bowl, mix together the butter and yogurt, then add to the dry mixture. Knead briefly and roll into 1 big ball. Halve the dough, then halve again, and keep halving until you have 16 lumps of dough. Roll into balls.

3. Place the balls of dough onto the prepared baking sheets and then flatten gently with the palm of your hand.

4. Bake for 15 minutes, or until the biscuits are cooked through and spring back from a firm touch. The biscuits may stay light in color.

5. Store leftovers, wrapped in aluminum foil or in an air-tight container, at room temperature for up to 5 days. Alternatively, freeze unbaked biscuit dough balls in freezer-safe bags for several months. Defrost at room temperature for 30 minutes before baking as described above.

6. Baked biscuits can also be frozen for up to 2 months. Defrost at room temperature for at least 1 hour. They can be eaten cold, but I prefer them warmed up in the toaster oven or in a 200°F oven for 5 to 10 minutes.

DESSERT

YOGURT OATMEAL COOKIES

Is this breakfast or dessert? The ingredient list suggests the former, but the taste is definitely the latter!

Makes 24 cookies. Six cookies, served over the course of a week, or at least split between 2 different days, provide the weekly dairy dose. If a nut flour is used, the cookies will help protect against tree nut allergies as well.

1 cup plain full-fat thick-style Greek yogurt
1 small egg
5 tablespoons plus 1 teaspoon butter, softened
½ teaspoon vanilla extract
¼ teaspoon ground cinnamon
¼ teaspoon salt
1 cup confectioners' sugar
1½ cups quick-cooking oatmeal (4 packages, if using instant)
⅓ cup desiccated coconut or ½ cup all-purpose flour or Homemade Nut Flour (page 135)
¾ cup chocolate chips (optional)

1. Preheat the oven to 350°F. Lightly grease two baking sheets with butter and set aside.

2. In a large bowl, mix together the yogurt, egg, butter, and vanilla. Add the cinnamon, salt, and sugar and stir well. Stir in the oatmeal and coconut until well incorporated. Fold in the chocolate chips.

3. Shape 24 small balls, approximately 1 inch in diameter, and place on the prepared baking sheets. Bake for 20 minutes, or until the top of the cookie springs back to the touch.

The cookie color will stay pale. Cool on wire racks for about 20 minutes, then serve.

4. Store leftovers in an airtight container at room temperature or in the refrigerator for up to 7 days. Alternatively, freeze weekly portions of baked cookies in freezer-safe plastic bags for up to 4 weeks. Defrost at room temperature for at least 1 hour before serving.

MILK SPICE CAKE

This moist cake has a delicious creamy taste that can be masked by the addition of spices if your child hates milk. For a chocolate alternative, use 5 teaspoons of cocoa powder in place of the spices. If you need to avoid eggs, leave them out; the texture will be slightly more crumbly and dense but yummy just the same.

Makes one 9 × 13-inch cake.

Serve ⅟₁₈ cake twice a week to provide the weekly dairy dose.

> 2 cups all-purpose flour
> 1 cup milk powder
> 1 cup confectioners' sugar
> ½ teaspoon baking soda
> 1 teaspoon baking powder
> 1 teaspoon ground nutmeg
> 1 teaspoon ground ginger
> 1 to 2 teaspoons ground cinnamon
> 1 teaspoon salt
> 1 cup oil
> 1 cup whole milk
> 1 teaspoon vanilla extract
> 2 eggs (optional)

1. Preheat the oven to 350°F. Butter a 9 × 13-inch cake pan and set aside.

2. In a large bowl, combine the flour, milk powder, sugar, baking soda, baking powder, nutmeg, ginger, cinnamon, and salt. In a medium bowl, whisk together the oil, milk, vanilla, and if using, the eggs. Add the oil-milk mixture to the bowl with the dry ingredients. Mix until just combined; don't worry if the batter is a bit lumpy. Pour the batter into the prepared pan. Bake for 45 minutes, or until a toothpick inserted in the middle comes out clean.

3. Allow the cake to cool completely, for about 2 hours, and then slice into 18 even pieces, roughly 3 × 2 inches in size.

4. Store leftovers, covered, at room temperature for up to 5 days, or freeze for up to 2 months. Defrost at room temperature for at least 3 hours before serving.

Recipes for Wheat Allergy Prevention

Wheat	Weekly Amount
Weetabix, Large	2 biscuits
Weetabix, Bite Size	⅔ cup
Wheat Chex	¾ cup
Plain Whole Wheat Bread, Thin Slices	2 slices
Plain Whole Wheat Bread, Thick Slices	½ slice
Plain Whole Wheat Pita Bread	1 6-inch pita, weighing 1.75 ounces (50 g)
Pasta or Couscous (100% wheat)	1.5 ounces or 40 grams, uncooked (see below)
Pasta	Weekly Amount (40 grams, uncooked)
Macaroni	½ cup
Spaghetti	44 sticks
Fusilli	½ cup
Couscous	¼ cup

Weekly doses are the *minimum* a baby or child is currently advised to eat. It is fine, perhaps even desirable, to surpass the required amounts. It is also best if the baby or child is *exposed to each allergen at least twice a week, no matter the amount eaten the first day.* So if your child wolfs down 1 whole grain sandwich, using thinly sliced bread, on Monday, you still need to make sure she eats at least ½ sandwich (or ½ dose from a different wheat category) later in the week.

WHEAT FOR BABY

In addition to using some of the recipes below, try pureeing cooked pasta or soaking whole wheat bread in milk till mushy for easy-peasy wheat doses for the tiny baby. Older babies often like couscous as well.

Older babies may also like Weetabix. This whole grain wheat cereal is a national favorite in the United Kingdom. Think Wheat Chex meets Shredded Wheat: big biscuits of fine wheat strands. Soaked in milk, it starts becoming mushy immediately. My babies, once teething, often liked chewing on a dry Weetabix biscuit right from the box. If you can't find Weetabix in your cereal aisle, try Amazon.com or another online retailer.

WHEATY PORRIDGE JAMBALAYA

This recipe is an allergy-fighting powerhouse, battling five major allergies at once. Serve it at least twice a week, and you can consider your baby well protected from most food allergies. And it doesn't taste half bad! If your baby gobbles it up, make it in bulk and freeze individual portions for use over the next several weeks.

Makes about 1⅔ cups. The full recipe provides the weekly wheat, egg, sesame, peanut, and dairy doses, best served over 2 or more days.

⅔ cup full-fat milk
2 Weetabix biscuits or ¾ cup Wheat Chex
1 small hard-boiled egg
3 teaspoons tahini, well stirred
3 rounded teaspoons peanut butter

1. Heat the milk in a large microwave-safe bowl for about 2 minutes on high power in the microwave. Add the Weetabix. Allow the wheat cereal to completely soak up the milk, 10 to 15 minutes, and then stir until a smooth puree consistency is formed.

2. While you are waiting for the cereal to finish soaking, chop the egg. Place it in a small bowl and blend with 2 tablespoons water.

3. Add the blended egg paste, peanut butter, and tahini to the porridge, stirring well until completely combined. Stir in additional water, if needed, to get the consistency that is right for your baby. Serve warm.

4. Store leftovers in the refrigerator for up to 2 days, or freeze for 1 month. Defrost in the fridge for at least 5 hours and then reheat in the microwave or on the stovetop until piping hot.

TIP: If you desire, you can try mixing three or four of the key foods together first (like Weetabix-milk-tahini or Weetabix-milk-egg) before trying the full recipe. You may also add a bit of mashed banana or other pureed fruit to this recipe to give a hint of natural sweetness and added flavor.

MEALS AND SNACKS

WEETABIX BANANA MUFFINS

I developed this recipe as a nod to Dr. Lack's home country where, as I have mentioned, they love their Weetabix! If you can't find Weetabix, substitute ⅓ cup Wheat Chex for every large Weetabix biscuit.

**Makes 12 small muffins. Eight muffins, served over
the course of a week, provide the weekly wheat
dose; 6 will satisfy the egg and dairy doses.**

3 large Weetabix or 1 cup Wheat Chex
1⅓ cup whole milk
1 ripe banana
2 small eggs, beaten
½ teaspoon vanilla
1 cup sugar
1 cup flour
2 teaspoons baking powder
1 teaspoon ground cinnamon

1. Preheat the oven to 350°F. Lightly grease a 12-cup muffin pan with butter.

2. In a large bowl, pour the milk over the crushed wheat biscuits and mash in the banana. Mix in the eggs, vanilla, and sugar. Add the flour, baking powder, and cinnamon and mix until just combined; don't worry if the batter is lumpy.

3. Divide the batter among the muffin cups, filling two-thirds of the way, and bake for 25 to 35 minutes, until a toothpick inserted into the middle comes out clean.

4. Store leftovers in an airtight container at room temperature for up to 5 days, or freeze for up to 2 months. Defrost at room temperature for at least 30 minutes before serving.

BREAD CRUMB PRIMER

Using whole grain bread crumbs in meatballs and meat loaf, to coat fish and chicken tenders, or to make Faux-Fried Cheese Fingers (page 171) can be an excellent way to make whole grain wheat palatable to a sensitive child.

Makes 6 cups fresh bread crumbs or about 4 cups toasted bread crumbs. Serve ¾ cup fresh or ½ cup dry-toasted crumbs to provide the weekly wheat dose. It is best served over 2 or more days.

8 slices whole grain bread
1 teaspoon salt
½ teaspoon freshly ground black pepper
¼ teaspoon garlic powder

1. Place the bread in a food processor. Add salt, pepper, and garlic powder. Pulse to desired fineness.

2. The bread crumbs can be used fresh or toasted. To toast, spread on ungreased baking sheets and toast until dry, about 15 minutes, in a 450°F oven.

3. Store leftovers in an airtight container. Fresh crumbs, stored in the refrigerator, will last about 3 days. Well-toasted crumbs will last a month and should be stored at room temperature.

NEAT WHEAT SLIDERS OR MEAT "BREADSTICKS"

This recipe hides egg and wheat among ground beef in the shape of small round burger patties ("sliders") or long sausage shapes ("breadsticks"). I often make 12 of each shape and give the kids a choice. Grant likes to dip the breadsticks in ketchup, whereas Clara likes to top the sliders with cottage cheese and tuck them into a bit of pita bread.

Makes 24 sliders or "breadsticks."
One-quarter of the recipe, served over the course of
a week, provides the weekly egg and wheat doses.

4 small eggs
14 ounces (400 g) lean ground steak
4 slices of whole wheat bread, crumbed
   (see Bread Crumb Primer on page 186)
½ teaspoon salt
¼ teaspoon freshly ground black pepper
¼ teaspoon garlic granules
¼ teaspoon smoked paprika
⅓ cup finely grated Parmesan (optional)

1. Preheat the oven to 450°F. Grease three baking sheets with olive or vegetable oil or butter. (If, like most people, you have only two baking sheets, make the recipe in two batches, refrigerating the first batch for a quick meal later in the week and serving the second batch straight from the oven.)

2. Combine all the ingredients in a large bowl, mixing well with clean hands. For the sliders, roll the mixture into 2- to 3-inch balls and then gently flatten them with a spatula or your hand on the prepared baking sheet. For the breadsticks, roll small portions of the mixture into 4-inch-long sticklike shapes. Bake until browned, about 25 minutes.

3. Store leftovers wrapped in plastic in the refrigerator for up to 3 days. Reheat thoroughly in the microwave or on a skillet over medium-low heat. Alternatively, place in a 200°F oven for about 10 minutes (flipping halfway), before serving. The texture of the leftovers will be a bit softer, especially if you use a microwave to reheat, but my children have never seemed to be bothered. Alternatively, you can freeze the leftovers for up to 2 months. Defrost overnight in the fridge and then reheat as described above before serving.

COUSCOUS-COATED CHICKEN

Golden and delectable—I had to ask my husband to save some for the kids! For variation, and to fight fish or dairy allergies simultaneously, you could try subbing fish or halloumi cheese for the chicken, decreasing the baking time to 20 minutes.

Makes about 4 servings.
One-quarter of the recipe provides the weekly
wheat dose, best served over 2 or more days.

1 cup uncooked couscous
¼ teaspoon salt
1 cup boiling water
1 cup all-purpose flour
½ teaspoon salt
½ teaspoon freshly ground black pepper
15 ounces (425 g) of boneless, skinless chicken,
    cut into strips
1 egg
2 tablespoons whole milk

1. Preheat the oven to 425°F. Thickly coat two baking sheets with olive or vegetable oil and set aside.

2. Put the couscous and salt in a deep bowl. Add the boiling water, stir once, and cover for at least 5 minutes. Set aside.

3. In a wide, shallow bowl or pie pan, beat together the egg and the milk.

4. Put the flour in another wide, shallow bowl and stir in seasonings, mixing well. Dredge the chicken strips in the flour mixture and stir until all pieces are well coated.

5. Fluff the couscous with a fork so that there are no remaining clumps. Working piece by piece, shake the excess flour off the chicken and submerge in the egg mixture, then in the couscous. Place the coated chicken strips on the prepared baking sheets.

6. Bake for at least 30 minutes, flipping once, until chicken is cooked through and the couscous is lightly golden.

7. Store leftovers in an airtight container in the refrigerator for up to 4 days, or freeze for up to 6 months. Bake from frozen in a 425°F oven for 25 minutes, or until piping hot.

DESSERT

WEETABIX PEANUT BUTTER CHOCOLATE CHIP COOKIES

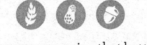

Another yummy, scrummy recipe that battles several allergies in one go. You can sub in any type of nut butter or flour. If you don't have nut flour around, using just all-purpose flour will be fine, though you won't get the same amount of nut protection. The chocolate chips aren't really necessary, but if you want to do some serious allergy preventing, the chocolate does make them particularly addictive.

Makes 24 small cookies.
Six cookies, served over the course of a week, provide the weekly wheat dose; 3 cookies in a week provide the weekly peanut dose; and 6 or more cookies in a week could help prevent some tree nut allergies.

4 large Weetabix or 1⅓ cups Wheat Chex
8 tablespoons (1 stick) butter, softened
½ cup peanut butter
⅓ cup granulated sugar
⅓ cup (packed) light or dark brown sugar
½ cup almond or other tree nut flour (see Homemade Nut Flour, on page 135, to make your own)
½ cup all-purpose flour
½ cup chocolate chips (optional)

1. Preheat the oven to 350°F.

2. Crush the Weetabix until fine. To do this, either use the pulse function on a food processor, or my kids' favorite, place in a resealable plastic bag and pound with rolling pin or ice cream scooper. Set aside.

3. Cream together the butter, peanut butter, and sugars in a large bowl or the bowl of your mixer. Mix until the combination is uniform; there will be a slight grainy consistency. Stir in the flours until well combined and the mixture resembles, well, cookie dough. Stir in the chocolate chips.

4. Form the dough into 1-inch balls and place on two ungreased baking sheets. (At this stage, you may freeze the unbaked cookie dough balls for up to 3 months.) Press the balls down to flatten ever so slightly before popping into the oven.

5. Bake for 20 to 25 minutes, until the cookies' surfaces lose their shine and the batter has set. Allow to cool for at least 45 minutes. Don't worry if they seem overly crumbly while still hot. They have a perfect texture once cool.

6. Frozen cookie dough balls may be baked straight from the freezer in a 350°F oven for 25 to 30 minutes.

7. Store in an airtight container at room temperature for up to 7 days, or freeze baked cookies for up to 3 months. Defrost at room temperature for at least 1 hour before serving.

SESAME COOKIES

This delicate cookie is the type I crave alongside a piping hot mug of Earl Grey. Light and yet, with the tahini and orange zest, deeply satisfying. I am not sure my kids spend the time savoring this complexity, however. They wolf the cookie down before I can even pour them a glass of milk to go with it!

**Makes 12 cookies. Five cookies provide
the weekly wheat and sesame doses.**

4 tablespoons (½ stick) butter, softened
¼ cup sugar
2½ tablespoons tahini, well stirred
½ teaspoon vanilla extract
¼ teaspoon ground cinnamon, plus ¼ teaspoon for dusting
¼ teaspoon grated orange zest or orange extract
Pinch of salt
¾ cup whole grain wheat flour
½ teaspoon baking powder
1 tablespoon confectioners' sugar, for dusting

1. Using a mixer on high speed, beat the butter and sugar in a large bowl until fluffy and creamy, about 6 minutes. Lower the speed and add the tahini, vanilla, cinnamon, orange zest, and salt. Mix to a smooth consistency. Add the flour and baking powder until the dough is smooth. Cover and refrigerate for 1 hour.

2. Preheat the oven to 350°F. Line a baking sheet with parchment paper and set aside.

3. To dust the dough, mix the confectioners' sugar and cinnamon in a small bowl. Take pieces of dough and form balls the size of large olives. Roll the balls in the sugar-cinnamon mixture and place on the prepared baking sheet, spacing them about ½ inch apart. Bake for 15 to 20 minutes. The cookies should set but still be light colored when done. To avoid breakage, don't move them until they are completely cool.

4. Store leftovers in an airtight container at room temperature for up to 7 days, or freeze, in between layers of parchment paper, in a freezer-safe container for up to 6 weeks. Defrost at room temperature for at least 1 hour before serving.

Recipes for Fish Allergy Prevention

Fish	Weekly Amount
Fresh/Frozen Fish	¼ 3.5-ounce fillet (about 25 g)
Fish Sticks	2 average fish sticks
Canned Fish	About 0.8 ounces (25 g), drained

Types of Fish to Embrace	
White Fish	Oily
Cod	Salmon
Flounder	Mackerel
Sole	Herring
Pollack	Pilchard
Haddock	Sardine
Plaice	Trout

Weekly doses are the *minimum* a baby or child is currently advised to eat. It is fine, perhaps even desirable, to surpass the required amounts. It is also best if the baby or child is *exposed to each allergen at least twice a week, no matter the amount eaten the first day.* So if your child wolfs down 2 fish sticks on Monday, you still need to make sure she eats at least $^1/_8$ of a 3.5-ounce fish fillet (or ½ dose from a different fish category) later in the week.

FISH FOR BABY

BASIC FISH
PUREE

All three of my babies have *loved* this! Which is probably why I always have made it in bulk. It freezes well and defrosts quickly—perfect for when your baby suddenly decides he needs dinner now!

Makes about 3 cups.
This recipe makes 16 weekly fish or shellfish doses.

2 medium sweet or white starchy potatoes,
   such as Idaho russet
14 ounces (400 g) skinless, boneless fish or shellfish,
   such as salmon, cod, haddock, crab, or shrimp
1½ cups chopped vegetables, such as broccoli,
   zucchini, tomatoes, green beans, anything!

1. Preheat the oven to 375°F. Coat a 10 × 14-inch roasting pan with 2 tablespoons olive oil and set aside.

2. Scrub, peel, and dice the potatoes into 1-inch cubes. Don't labor over the shape; you will puree later. Place the potatoes on the prepared pan and place in the oven. Bake for 25 minutes, then add the fish and vegetables to the pan with the potatoes. Bake for another 20 minutes, or until the fish is cooked through and the vegetables are tender. Remove from the oven and let cool for 5 to 10 minutes, until easy to handle.

3. Place all the ingredients in a large food processor. Blend to desired consistency, adding water to thin if necessary.

4. Divide the mixture into individual servings (the size of which will depend on the age of your baby) in freezer-safe baby food containers. Serve your baby one portion within the next 24 hours, and freeze the rest for use over the next month. Defrost in the fridge for 4 to 6 hours and then reheat thoroughly in a microwave or on the stovetop before serving.

BABY'S FIRST FISH PIE

Fish and meat pies are very popular in England, where the EAT study was conducted. This freezable recipe uses many of the key ingredients for a fish pie but does not fuss about with putting them together into a proper savory pie. Instead, the ingredients are simply mashed or pureed together, making a well-rounded and allergy-fighting meal for baby.

Makes about eight ¼-cup servings.
This recipe makes 4 weekly fish doses and 1 weekly dairy dose.

⅔ cup whole milk
3.5 ounces (100 g) white or oily fish, such as cod or salmon
1 medium potato, scrubbed, peeled, and chopped
    (about 1 cup)
⅓ cup fresh or frozen peas
Sprinkle of minced fresh parsley or dried (optional)

1. Pour the milk into a wide saucepan, add the fish, and cook over medium-low heat for about 10 minutes, until the cooked fish flakes easily. Take out the fish and remove any bones and skin. Set aside.

2. Pour the cooking liquid through a fine-mesh sieve and return the strained liquid to the pan. Cook the potato pieces in this liquid over medium-low heat until they are soft, 15 to 20 minutes.

3. Stir in the peas and, if using, the parsley and cook for 1 additional minute over medium-low heat. Turn off the heat and add the fish back to the pot.

4. In a medium bowl, mash together the ingredients with the back of a fork (or puree in a blender or food processor or use an immersion blender) until the mixture becomes the consistency that suits your baby.

5. Divide the finished puree into four equal ½-cup portions. Store one in the refrigerator for use within the next 2 days.

6. Freeze the remaining three portions for up to 3 months. Defrost overnight in the fridge and then reheat thoroughly in a microwave or a pot over medium heat before serving.

NUTTY FISH PUREE OR SPREAD

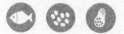

This versatile multitasking recipe fights at least three allergies at once. You could experiment with adding additional nut butters to fight more nut allergies. For younger babies, mixing this puree with mashed sweet potato can make it a full and tasty meal. For teething babies and toddlers, try spreading on whole grain toast or tucking it in whole wheat pita bread to meet the wheat quota as well.

Makes 2 servings.
The full recipe provides the weekly fish, sesame,
and peanut doses. It is best served
2 or more times over the week.

0.9 ounces (25 g) freshly cooked or canned tuna or salmon
3 teaspoons tahini, well stirred
3 rounded teaspoons smooth peanut butter

1. In a small bowl, mash the tuna with 1 tablespoon water, using a fork (or puree in a blender). Mix the tahini and peanut butter into the mashed tuna. If needed, add another tablespoon of water to the mixture, stirring or blending until a smooth pastelike consistency is reached. Serve cold or warm, as your baby prefers. To warm, microwave at full power for 15 to 30 seconds and stir before serving.

2. Store leftovers in an airtight container in the refrigerator for up to 2 days. Alternatively, make the recipe in bulk and freeze in weekly portions for use over the next 2 months. Defrost in the fridge for 4 to 5 hours before serving.

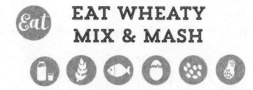

EAT WHEATY
MIX & MASH

If you are looking for the simplest way to protect your child from common food allergies, this is it. All the major food allergies studied in the EAT study are addressed by this recipe. Make the below and make sure your baby eats all of it over at least 2 days, every week. Job done.

Makes two to three rounded ½-cup servings.
The full recipe provides the weekly dairy, wheat,
fish, egg, sesame, and peanut doses.

⅔ cup whole milk
2 Weetabix biscuits or ¾ cup Wheat Chex
0.9 ounces (25 g) cooked fish, such as cod, haddock,
    or salmon
1 small hard-boiled egg
3 teaspoons tahini, well stirred
3 rounded teaspoons peanut butter

1. Heat the milk in a small microwave-safe bowl for 1 to 2 minutes on high power in the microwave or in a small heavy-bottomed pot over medium-low heat until steaming. Pour into a small soup or cereal bowl. Add the Weetabix biscuits and allow the cereal to soak up the milk for at least 15 minutes.

2. While the cereal is soaking, blend together the fish and egg in a food processor or blender, adding water to make it a smooth paste. Scrape the paste into a large microwave-safe bowl and stir in the soaked cereal until it resembles a smooth porridge. Next stir in the tahini and peanut butter until it disappears into the porridge. (This is easiest to do if the porridge is still warm. If it has cooled, reheat it for 30 seconds on medium power in the microwave or for a minute or two in a saucepan on the stovetop over medium-low heat.)

Add the blended egg-fish mixture. Stir in a tablespoon or more of water if the consistency is too thick for your infant.

3. Store leftovers in an airtight container in the refrigerator for up to 2 days. Alternatively, make the above in bulk and freeze in weekly portions for use over the next 3 months. Defrost in the fridge for 4 to 5 hours and then reheat in the microwave or in a pot over medium heat, stirring often, until piping hot.

TIP: If desired, you may also add a bit of mashed sweet potato, banana, or other pureed fruit to give a hint of natural sweetness and added flavor. As your baby gets older, mix in well-flaked fish or mashed ripe pieces of fruit to offer a lumpier texture.

VARIATION: Make Kiwi EAT Wheaty Mix & Mash by blending a kiwi in the food processor with the fish and egg. To up the allergy-fighting prowess of this recipe even further, try adding cooked shrimp to the blender and other nut butters, such as almond butter or cashew butter or a home-made mixture (see page 133).

LUNCH/DINNER/SNACK

SALMON, BROCCOLI, AND CHEESE PASTA

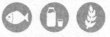

A healthful, toddler-friendly meal that just happens to battle three potential food allergies at once! I often triple the amounts and feed the whole family.

Makes four ½-cup toddler-size servings.
The full recipe provides 4 weekly fish doses, 2 weekly dairy doses, and 1 weekly wheat dose. One portion, a quarter of the entire recipe, will provide the weekly fish dose, half the weekly dairy dose, and a quarter of the weekly wheat dose.

> 3.5 ounces (100 g) salmon
> ½ cup uncooked fusilli or macaroni
> 4 to 8 broccoli florets
> 1 tablespoon butter
> ⅔ cup whole milk
> 1 tablespoon all-purpose flour
> 2 tablespoons grated cheddar cheese

1. Preheat the oven to 400°F.

2. Thickly coat a 9 × 13-inch baking sheet with olive or vegetable oil. Place the salmon on the baking sheet and pop into the oven. Remove after about 15 minutes, when the salmon is cooked through and is a uniform light pink both inside and out. Set aside.

3. Bring a large pot of water to a boil, add the pasta, and cook about 10 to 11 minutes. After the first 5 minutes, place the broccoli in a sieve over the pasta and allow to steam. Alternatively, place the broccoli in a small microwave-safe bowl, add 2 to 3 tablespoons of water, cover with a microwave-safe plate, and microwave on medium power for 1 to 3 minutes, until the broccoli is tender.

4. While the pasta is cooking, make a cheese sauce by melting the butter over medium-low heat in a small saucepan. Whisk in the milk and flour, stirring over medium-low heat until the mixture thickens. Add the grated cheese and stir until thoroughly melted and combined. Drain the pasta and broccoli and place in a serving dish. Break up the salmon into bite-size pieces and add to the serving dish. Pour the sauce over and serve.

5. Store leftovers in an airtight container in the refrigerator for up to 3 days, or freeze for use over the next 2 months. Defrost in the fridge for 3 to 4 hours and then reheat thoroughly in a microwave or stove pot over medium heat. Stir before serving.

SALMON-SHRIMP SLIDERS

You can use cooked or raw salmon and shrimp in this feed-the-whole-family recipe. I prefer cooked as it makes the last, predinner step faster, and it is easiest to peel the skin off simply baked salmon. But you can also skip the roasting step altogether and go straight to the food processor with raw fish.

Note: Honey may contain bacteria that can't be handled by the digestive system of a child less than one year old, so recipes containing honey should not be served to babies.

Makes 24 sliders.
Two sliders, served over the course of a week,
provide the weekly fish dose and may help protect from
shellfish allergy, too. To fight dairy allergy simultaneously,
these are good topped with a bit of Greek yogurt thinned
with orange juice. Try adding wasabi to the yogurt
topping for the grown-ups. Serve on whole wheat buns,
and you can check off 1 weekly wheat dose as well.

3 tablespoons of olive or vegetable oil
3 small skinless salmon fillets
    (about 11.6 ounces or 330 g total)
10 ounces (285 g) shelled shrimp
2 tablespoons honey
1 large egg
2 tablespoons pickled ginger (optional)
⅛ teaspoon salt
⅛ teaspoon freshly ground black pepper

1. Preheat the oven to 400°F.

2. Coat a baking sheet with 1 tablespoon of the oil. Put the fillets on the baking sheet skin side up. Bake for 10 minutes and then add the raw shrimp to the pan. Cook for another 5 to 10 minutes until the shrimp are pink and the fillets are cooked through and are a uniform pink throughout. Allow the fish to cool for a few minutes before peeling off the skin.

3. Place the salmon, shrimp, honey, egg, ginger (if using), salt, and pepper in a food processor. Pulse until well mashed but still chunky. Divide the mixture into twenty-four equal portions and shape them into 3-inch patties. Shallow-fry in the remaining 2 tablespoons oil over medium heat in a heavy-bottomed fry pan until golden brown, about 3 minutes on each side, or 6 minutes if the salmon and shrimp were not precooked.

4. Alternatively, heat the oven to 450°F. Grease a 13 × 18-inch baking sheet with the remaining oil. Place the patties on the prepared sheet, 1 to 2 inches apart, and bake in the oven for 12 to 15 minutes, flipping halfway through.

5. Store leftovers in an airtight container in the refrigerator for up to 3 days, or freeze for up to 2 months. Defrost frozen fish sliders overnight in the fridge and then pan-fry over medium heat for 3 minutes on each side until piping hot.

OVEN-BAKED FISH STICKS

Fish sticks are loved by all three of my kids and so they feature weekly. (The only other foods they all seem to agree on at the moment fall into the fruit or dessert categories.) I have two versions, depending on how time poor or ambitious I am feeling. If I am low on time, the first recipe below, #1 Time-Crunch Fish Sticks, takes only about 10 minutes to prep. If I go the ambitious route, opting for #2 Super-Mama Fish Fingers, I'll make the sticks in bulk, freezing future dinner portions before the baking stage. Make sure to use fresh fish if you want to freeze them later.

Turmeric is a strange ingredient to see in a book for kids. It is quite bitter. Here I am using it purely for color. It gives the sticks that golden color that store-bought fish sticks have. Use sparingly and it won't be tasted.

#1 TIME-CRUNCH FISH STICKS

Makes about 10 fish sticks, or enough to
feed 2 adults and 2 children. One-half fish stick
(¼ fillet) provides the weekly fish dose. Using Homemade
Nut Flour (page 135) will likely help protect from nut
allergies. Using whole wheat bread crumbs offers some
marginal protection from wheat allergy development.

5 small fillets boneless, skinless white fish, such as cod,
    haddock, or tilapia (about 17.6 ounces or 500 g total)
1 cup Homemade Nut Flour (page 135) or store bought, or
    homemade toasted bread crumbs (see page 186) or store
    bought
1 tablespoon dried herbs, such as thyme, parsley, or
    marjoram (optional)
⅛ teaspoon ground turmeric (optional)
Salt and freshly ground black pepper

1. Preheat the oven to 400°F. Lightly grease two baking sheets with 1 to 2 tablespoons butter.

2. With a sharp knife, cut each fillet into two finger-friendly strips. This is easiest to do if the fish is still a bit frozen. If using frozen fish, allow to defrost fully before continuing with the directions below. Blot the fish strips gently with paper towels to remove excess water and set aside.

3. Place the flour in a wide, shallow bowl or pie pan and stir in the herbs and turmeric, if using. Season to taste with salt and pepper.

4. Dredge the fish in the crumbs and place on the prepared baking sheets, spaced at least 2 inches apart. (Crowding them together makes the coating soggy.) Bake for 10 to 15 minutes until the coating browns a bit. Serve warm.

5. Store leftovers in an airtight container in the refrigerator for up to 3 days. Reheat in a 300°F oven for about 10 minutes until piping hot.

TIP: Serve with Tahini-Honey Dip (page 160) or a yogurt dip to battle **sesame** or **dairy** allergies simultaneously.

#2 SUPER-MAMA FISH FINGERS

Makes 20 fish fingers, or enough to feed 4 adults
and 4 to 6 children. One-half fish stick (¼ fillet)
provides the weekly fish dose. Using Homemade Nut
Flour (page 135) will likely help protect from some nut
allergies. Using whole wheat bread crumbs offers some
marginal protection from wheat allergy development.

10 small fillets boneless, skinless white fish, such as cod,
    haddock, or tilapia (about 35 ounces or 1 kg total)
1 cup all-purpose flour
Salt and freshly ground black pepper
3 small eggs

**2 cups fine homemade toasted bread crumbs (see page 186)
or store bought
2 tablespoons dried herbs, such as thyme, parsley, or
marjoram (optional)
¼ teaspoon turmeric (optional)**

1. Preheat the oven to 400°F.

2. With a sharp knife, cut each fillet into two finger-friendly strips. Blot the fish strips gently with paper towels to remove excess water and set aside.

3. Set yourself up with one dinner plate and two wide, shallow bowls or pie pans. On the plate, spread the flour and season to taste with salt and pepper. In one pie pan, beat the eggs well. In the other pan, spread the bread crumbs and mix in the herbs and turmeric, if using. Season to taste with salt.

4. Working one by one, dredge the fish in the flour until completely coated and then dip into the egg mixture. Finally, roll in the bread crumbs. If freezing, do so at this stage (see Tip below). They will keep for up to 3 months.

5. When ready to cook, place the fish sticks at least 2 inches apart. (I find closer spacing leads to soggy coating.) Bake for 12 minutes, or 25 minutes if baking from frozen, until the coating is golden brown and the fish is cooked through. The fish should be firm and opaque in the middle. See Tip on page 208 for optional allergy-fighting sauces to serve alongside.

6. Store leftovers in an airtight container in the refrigerator for up to 3 days. Reheat from frozen in a 300°F oven for about 10 minutes until piping hot.

FREEZING TIP: I find it easiest to freeze on trays or whatever flat-surfaced item will fit in your freezer and then, once hard, to transfer to freezer bags or containers. Do not defrost before baking or the coating will become mushy.

PIZZA FISH

Kid-friendly, family-friendly fish beyond fish fingers! If you are defrosting fish for this recipe, cut them first before they thaw. Frozen fish is much easier to cut neatly than fresh or defrosted fillets. Allow the fish to thoroughly defrost before continuing with the recipe.

Makes about 8 "pizza fish," or enough to feed 2 adults and 2 to 4 children. The full recipe provides 16 weekly fish doses and 5½ weekly dairy doses. One "pizza fish" provides 2 weekly fish doses and more than ½ weekly dairy dose.

4 haddock fillets (about 14 ounces or 400 g)
1 cup finely grated Parmesan cheese
⅓ cup tomato sauce, pureed canned tomatoes, or pesto

1. Preheat the oven to 400°F. Coat a baking sheet with 1 to 2 tablespoons olive or vegetable oil and set aside.

2. Cut each fillet parallel to the countertop to make about ¾-inch thin and flat surfaces.

3. Blot the fillet slices with paper towels to remove excess water and place on the prepared baking sheet. Make "pizza fishes" by spreading each fillet slice with a spoonful of sauce and a generous amount of cheese.

4. Bake until toasty brown, with bubbling cheese, about 20 minutes.

5. Store in an airtight container in the refrigerator for up to 3 days. Reheat in a 200°F oven or toaster oven for 5 to 10 minutes. Don't freeze, especially if you defrosted fish to make this.

TUNA BOLOGNESE

A fishy spin on a kid staple, and they'll never guess there is fish in the sauce. You can also try replacing the tuna with ½ cooked cod fillet (about 1.75 ounces or 50 g).

Makes 2 small servings.
Each serving provides the weekly fish, dairy, and wheat doses.

3 ounces (80 g) uncooked spaghetti
1 tablespoon olive oil
1 small onion, chopped
½ tablespoon butter
1 garlic clove, minced
1 cup canned chopped tomatoes
½ teaspoon dried Italian herbs, such as oregano
   or basil (optional)
1 5-ounce can light tuna, packed in water
⅓ rounded cup finely grated Parmesan cheese,
   plus more for serving

1. Boil the spaghetti according to the directions on the package.

2. Heat the oil in a pan. Add the onion and sauté for 5 to 7 minutes, until softened. Add butter and garlic. Cook for 1 minute. Stir in the tomatoes and, if using, the herbs.

3. Drain the tuna and empty into a small bowl. Break up the chunks with a fork, then add to the onion and tomato mixture. Stir in the Parmesan until melted.

4. Pour the sauce over the drained pasta and mix so that each strand of spaghetti is well covered. Serve with additional Parmesan.

5. Store leftovers in the refrigerator for up to 3 days. Alternatively, make the sauce in bulk and freeze portions for use over the next 2 months.

COD BALLS AND PATTIES

These are very popular in my house among all the different age groups, including the grown-ups. They are a great make-ahead treat that store well in the freezer. Bake from frozen!

Makes about 20 balls and patties, or enough to feed 2 to 3 adults and 2 to 4 children. Two-thirds of a ball, eaten twice a week, will help protect from fish allergy. Five balls provide ¼ egg and, if using whole wheat bread crumbs, ½ the weekly wheat dose.

2 medium sweet potatoes (about ⅔ pound total), scrubbed, peeled, and quartered
1 medium onion, quartered
4 garlic cloves
Salt
14 ounces (400 g) fresh or defrosted cod loin
1 medium egg
½ teaspoon dried oregano
¼ teaspoon freshly ground black pepper
1 cup toasted homemade bread crumbs (see page 186)

1. Preheat the oven to 350°F. Coat two baking sheets with 1 to 2 tablespoons olive or vegetable oil and set aside.

2. Place the potatoes, onion, and garlic on one of the prepared baking sheets and bake until the potatoes are soft, about 45 minutes.

3. Salt both sides of the cod and place on the second prepared baking sheet. Bake until cooked through and flaky, 20 to 25 minutes.

4. Allow the vegetables and cod to cool slightly, then place in large food processor. Add the egg, oregano, and pepper and blend for about 1 minute, until well combined. You want to leave it a bit lumpy.

5. Shape 2-inch balls and 3-inch patties. I like to roll the balls in bread crumbs and leave the patties bare because my kids prefer naked patties. But you could mix it up and do some balls and patties with bread crumbs and some without, so there are lots of options to choose from. You can stop here and store covered in the refrigerator for up to 1 day, or if using fresh cod, freeze for up to 2 months. (Do not refreeze previously frozen cod.)

6. Preheat the oven to 400°F. Bake on an ungreased baking sheet for about 20 minutes (35 minutes if baking from frozen), until golden brown. Allow a choice between the shapes at the table. Serve with tomato sauce and, if you wish, a side of pasta.

7. Store leftovers in an airtight container in the refrigerator for up to 3 days. Reheat in a 300°F oven or toaster oven for 10 minutes.

Acknowledgments

I owe many, many thanks to Gideon Lack and the other EAT and LEAP study researchers for their assistance and materials, including the EAT study handbook and supplemental documents. I would particularly like to thank Joanna Craven, for her excellent explanations, and Bunmi Raji, the EAT study dietician.

I am indebted to the many researchers and nutritionists who took time out of their busy lives to chat, send journal articles, or otherwise share information with me, especially James Baker, Hugh Sampson, Ellyn Satter, and Whitney Block.

I would like to thank my agent, Michelle Tessler, for her immediate enthusiasm for this book idea and my original editor, Deborah Brody, and her assistant, Madeline Jaffe, for the helpful suggestions, comments, and guidance on the manuscript. I am also grateful for Cara Bedick's assistance and to my final editor, Cassie Jones, who turned the manuscript into a proper book. And, of course, a big thank you to William Morrow, for their interest from the start.

I am also grateful to Magdalena Drabik, who kept my household running, and my kids happy, on the days I needed to spend quality time with my computer.

Last but far from least, I owe a very special thanks to Clara, Grady, and Arthur for all their feedback and help developing the recipes. And I am grateful, most of all, to Will, for his support and encouragement every step of the way.

Appendix: Weekly Feeding Worksheets

Starting when your infant is three to four months old, and following appropriate testing, use the chart provided to track your baby's exposure to common allergens. Write the amount that your baby eats of each potential allergen every day, trying to reach the amounts recommended below, over at least two servings, by the end of each week. This will become easier as your baby grows! You may even find that allergen feeding becomes quite routine. This exposure should be continued through kindergarten.

I've included some additional potential allergens (tree nuts, kiwi, banana, soy, shellfish) that have not been adequately studied yet. For now, just aim for exposure, as much as you can, without causing you or your baby stress. If you need additional worksheets, please visit this book's page on my website, Robin NixonPompa.com.

Weekly Guidelines for Preventing Food Allergies

- 2 1.5-ounce (40 g) containers plain yogurt or dairy equivalent (full fat for children under two years old)

- 1 small egg

- 3 rounded teaspoons peanut butter (use smooth, not chunky, for babies) or 5 teaspoons ground peanuts

- 3 teaspoons tahini or sesame equivalent

- 0.9 ounce (25 g) fish (about ¼ of an adult serving)

- 1 slice of whole wheat bread or wheat equivalent

Worksheet

Week #	Monday	Tuesday	Wednesday	Thursday
Dairy				
Egg				
Fish				
Peanut				
Sesame				
Wheat				
Tree nuts				
Kiwi				
Banana				
Soy				
Shellfish				

Friday	Saturday	Sunday	Total

Resources and Support Networks

Many of these resources are for kids and parents of kids who already have some food allergies. But many also follow cutting-edge developments involving food allergies, whether it is scientific research, new policies, new guidelines, or new services.

For the Latest Research

Food Allergy Research and Education (FARE)
http://www.foodallergy.org/
One of the best places to receive helpful and up-to-date information, this organization provides a range of resources from handbooks for the newly diagnosed to information on how to participate in a clinical trial.

National Institute of Allergy and Infectious Diseases (NIAID)
https://www.niaid.nih.gov/topics/foodallergy/Pages/default.aspx
Part of the National Institutes of Health, this institute is supporting many cutting-edge developments in food allergy research. Its Food Allergy webpage is reader friendly, timely, and will appeal to both the newly diagnosed and hardened allergy sufferers.

For Advocacy and Community

Kids with Food Allergies
http://www.kidswithfoodallergies.org/
A division of the Asthma and Allergy Foundation of America that focuses on children and families, Kids with Food Allergies provides

educational resources for parents and schools as well as a free news-
letter and community forum.

Food Allergy and Anaphylaxis Connection Team (FAACT)

http://www.foodallergyawareness.org/
An organization dedicated to advocacy and awareness of allergies as well
as to connecting parents, teens, and children struggling with food allergies. Its overnight camps and teen activities are particularly inspired.

Centers for Disease Control and Prevention's Handbook for Preschools and Schools

*http://www.cdc.gov/healthyyouth/foodallergies/pdf/13_243135_A
_Food_Allergy_Web_508.pdf*
A 108-page handbook, ready to download, giving "voluntary guidelines for managing food allergies in schools and early care and education programs."

Talking with Kids about Allergies

http://kidshealth.org/en/kids/food-allergies.html
Sometimes kids listen better to an expert than they do to their own
parents, especially if the parents find themselves slipping into nag
mode! This article, which also has an audio edition, helps get vital
information across to even young children.

For Information on Participating in a Clinical Trial

World Health Organization's International Clinical Trials Registry

http://apps.who.int/trialsearch/default.aspx/
Type in "food allergy" and the name of your country into the search
engine, and you will be given a selection of clinical trials currently
recruiting participants.

Consortium of Food Allergy Research (CoFAR)

http://www.cofargroup.org
Funded by the National Institutes of Health, CoFAR is conducting
multicenter clinical and observational studies to advance our understanding of food allergies. The website includes tools that help predict whether a baby is likely to "grow out" of an egg or milk allergy.
See also **Food Allergy Research and Education (FARE)** on page 221.

To Donate to Further Research

Ending Allergies Together (EAT)

http://endallergiestogether.com

An organization completely devoted to raising money for and funding research on ending food allergies. You can donate directly, or shop through Amazon Smile to have 0.5 percent of eligible purchases go to research on food allergies.

For Information on Often-Related Health Issues

National Eczema Association

https://nationaleczema.org/eczema/child-eczema/

An organization dedicated to improving the lives of eczema sufferers by providing medically informed education and treatment tips. The group also helps fund research and serves as a conduit to clinical trials focusing on eczema.

Asthma and Allergy Foundation of America (AAFA)

http://www.aafa.org/page/asthma.aspx

This not-for-profit organization provides valuable and up-to-date information on asthma (and allergies); it also funds research and helps connect people to local support groups.

United States Environmental Protection Agency (EPA)

https://www.epa.gov/asthma/publications-about-asthma#tab-1

This agency has a wealth of information on asthma and common triggers. It also publishes fun kid-focused books on learning to live with asthma.

The British Psychological Society; Living with Severe Food Allergy

https://thepsychologist.bps.org.uk/volume-27/edition-5/living-severe -food-allergy

Important information on the psychological strain of food allergies on both parents and children. The site includes an audio interview with a scientist who began researching the subject after her young son was diagnosed with a food allergy.

Foods and Supplies

Nuts.com

https://nuts.com/cookingbaking/flours/
This online retailer and international shipper obviously sells nuts but also finely ground nut flours (including soy) and almond, cashew, and peanut butters.

Artisana Organics

http://www.artisanaorganics.com/
While peanut butter can be found almost anywhere, other nut butters are harder to locate. Artisana, sold through Amazon and other retailers, makes pecan, walnut, and other less available nut butters.

Food Processors

https://www.cuisinart.com/products/food_processors.html
If you can find room in your kitchen and budget, I highly recommend buying the largest and highest-quality food processor you can afford. They are invaluable for making purees, nut flours and butters, and whole wheat bread crumbs, thus making essential allergens palatable to babies and kids. My six-year-old Cuisinart, or the sous-chef, as I call her, has processed baby food for three kids, makes near constant supplies of mixed-nut butter, and even helps my husband make Bolognese on occasion. I am not sure what we would do without her! (That said, at the end of 2016, Cuisinart recalled 8 million food processors, sold between 1996 and 2015, due to a laceration hazard. So do your research before buying!)

Universal Conversion Chart

Oven Temperature Equivalents

250°F = 120°C
275°F = 135°C
300°F = 150°C
325°F = 160°C
350°F = 180°C
375°F = 190°C
400°F = 200°C
425°F = 220°C
450°F = 230°C
475°F = 240°C
500°F = 260°C

Measurement Equivalents

Measurements should always be level unless directed otherwise.

⅛ teaspoon = 0.5 mL
¼ teaspoon = 1 mL
½ teaspoon = 2 mL
1 teaspoon = 5 mL
1 tablespoon = 3 teaspoons = ½ fluid ounce = 15 mL
2 tablespoons = ⅛ cup = 1 fluid ounce = 30 mL
4 tablespoons = ¼ cup = 2 fluid ounces = 60 mL
5⅓ tablespoons = ⅓ cup = 3 fluid ounces = 80 mL
8 tablespoons = ½ cup = 4 fluid ounces = 120 mL
10⅔ tablespoons = ⅔ cup = 5 fluid ounces = 160 mL
12 tablespoons = ¾ cup = 6 fluid ounces = 180 mL
16 tablespoons = 1 cup = 8 fluid ounces = 240 mL

Notes

Introduction

1   Trisha remembers three-year-old Henry's babyhood: Trisha Woodfire, mother of formerly food-allergic Henry, in discussion with the author, June 4, 2015. Names changed by request.

4   an increased risk of food allergies due to her brother's condition: Hui-Ju Tsai, Rajesh Kumar, Jacqueline Pongracic, Xin Liu, Rachel Story, Yunxian Yu, Deanna Caruso, et al,, "Familial Aggregation of Food Allergy and Sensitization to Food Allergens: A Family-Based Study," *Clinical and Experimental Allergy* 39 (2009): 101–9, doi:10.1111/j.1365-2222.2008.03111.x.

4   Autoimmune diseases and allergies are both on the rise: Hikaru Okada, Chantal Kuhn, Hélène Feillet, and Jean-François Bach, "The 'Hygiene Hypothesis' for Autoimmune and Allergic Diseases: An Update," *Clinical and Experimental Immunology* 160 (2010): 1–9; and Stefan Ehlars and Stefan H. E. Kaufman, "Infection, Inflammation, and Chronic Diseases: Consequences of a Modern Lifestyle," *Trends in Immunology* 31, no. 5 (2010): 184–90, doi:10.1016/j.it.2010.02.003.

5   When Ben was Oliver's age: Pippa George, mother of food-allergic Ben and Oliver, in discussion with the author, May 21, 2015.

7   but research has shown it does not: Michael R. Perkin, Kirsty Logan, Anna Tseng, Bunmi Raji, Salma Ayis, Janet Peacock, Helen Brough, et al., "Randomized Trial of Introduction of Allergenic Foods in Breast-Fed Infants," *New England Journal of Medicine* 374 (2016): 1733–43, doi:10.1056/NEJMoa1514210.

13   the EAT study researchers gave participants a handbook: "Early Introduction Group, Follow On Tips and Recipes, Version 3." Courtesy of Enquiring About Tolerance (EAT) study researchers.

http://www.eatstudy.co.uk/wp-content/uploads/2010/10/FollowOn Booklet_version3updated.pdf. Last updated March 17, 2011.

Chapter 1: The Problem

17   an estimated 6 to 8 percent of children: Scott H. Sicherer and Hugh A. Sampson, "Food Allergy: Epidemiology, Pathogenesis, Diagnosis, and Treatment," *Journal of Allergy and Clinical Immunology* 133, no. 2 (2014): 291–307, http://www.jacionline.org/article/S0091 –6749(13)01836–8/pdf.

17   one in ten preschool children in developed countries: Susan L. Prescott, Ruby Pawankar, Katrina J. Allen, Dianne E. Campbell, John K. H. Sinn, Alessandro Fiocchi, Motohiro Ebisawa, et al., "A Global Survey of Changing Patterns of Food Allergy Burden in Children." *World Allergy Organization Journal* 6 (2013): 21, http://www .waojournal.org/content/6/1/21.

17   Every three minutes: Sunday Clark, Janice Espinola, Susan A. Rudders, Aleena Banerji, and Carlos A. Camargo Jr., "Frequency of US Emergency Department Visits for Food-Related Acute Allergic Reactions," *Journal of Allergy and Clinical Immunology* 127, no. 3 (2011): 682–83. Cited by FARE statistics.

18   They rose 50 percent: Kristen D. Jackson, LaJeana D. Howie, and Lara J. Akinbami, "Trends in Allergic Conditions Among Children: United States, 1997–2011." NCHS Data Brief no. 121. National Center for Health Statistics, Hyattsville, MD, May 2013, http://www.ncbi .nlm.nih.gov/pubmed/23742874.

18   the prevalence of food allergy had doubled: Allergy UK, "Allergy Statistics," 2016. Citing the European Academy of Allergy and Clinical Immunology, 2015, https://www.allergyuk.org/allergy -statistics/allergy-statistics.

18   increased psychological issues: Mary D. Klinnert and Jane L. Robinson, "Addressing the Psychological Needs of Families of Food-Allergic Children," *Current Allergy and Asthma Reports* 8 (2008): 195–200.

18   "atopic march": Katrina J. Allen and Jennifer J. Koplin, "Theories on the Increasing Prevalence of Food Allergy," in *Food Allergy: Adverse Reactions to Foods and Food Additives*, 5th ed., eds. Dean D. Metcalfe, Hugh A. Sampson, Ronald A. Simon, and Gideon Lack

(New York: John Wiley, 2014), 123–33; and Michael R. Perkin, Kirsty Logan, Tom Marrs, Suzana Radulovic, Joanna Craven, Carsten Flohr, and Gideon Lack on behalf of the EAT Study Team, "Enquiring About Tolerance (EAT) Study: Feasibility of an Early Allergenic Food Introduction Regimen," *Journal of Allergy and Clinical Immunology* 137, no. 5 (2016): 1477–86. http://dx.doi.org/10.1016/j.jaci.2015.12.1322.

18   nearly six million kids in the United States: Ruchi S. Gupta, Elizabeth E. Springston, Manoj R. Warrier, Bridget Smith, Rajesh Kumar, Jacqueline Pongracic, and Jane L. Holl, "The Prevalence, Severity, and Distribution of Childhood Food Allergy in the United States," *Pediatrics* 128, no. 1 (2011): e9-e17, doi:10.1542/peds.2011-0204.

18   one million in the United Kingdom: Allergy UK, "Allergy Statistics," 2016. Citing the National Institute for Health and Clinical Excellence, 2011, https://www.allergyuk.org/allergy-statistics/allergy-statistics.

20   Mithridatism, as the strategy is still sometimes called: *Wikipedia*, s.v. "Mithridatism," last modified March 2016, https://en.wikipedia.org/wiki/Mithridatism.

20   the legendary "arsenic eaters of Styria": "The Arsenic Eaters of Styria," *Scientific American*, October 2, 1869, accessed March 24, 2015, http://www.scientificamerican.com/article/the-arsenic-eaters-of-styria/.

22   oral immunotherapy is being explored: Jay S. Skyler. "Toward Primary Prevention of Type 1 Diabetes," *Journal of the American Medical Association* 313, no. 15 (2015): 1520–21; and Kendra Vehik, David Cuthbertson, Holly Ruhlig, Desmond A. Schatz, Mark Peakman, and Jeffrey P. Krischer, "DPT-1 and TrialNet Study Groups. Long-Term Outcome of Individuals Treated with Oral Insulin: Diabetes Prevention Trial-Type 1 (DPT-1) Oral Insulin Trial," *Diabetes Care* 34, no. 7 (2011): 1585–90.

23   vaccinations against food allergies: Rudolf Valenta, Heidrun Hochwallner, Birgit Linhart, and Sandra Pahr, "Food Allergies: The Basics," *Gastroenterology* 148, no. 6 (2015): 1120–31, http://dx.doi.org/10.1053/j.gastro.2015.02.006.

23   Deelan, who is seven: Harsha Rama, mother of two food-allergic children, in discussion with the author, June–July 2015.

26   "a fundamental change in the human immune system": James Baker, CEO and chief medical officer of Food Allergy Research and Education, in discussion with the author, March 29, 2016.

26   Peanuts and tree nuts are considered: Sabrina Bachai, "Food Allergy Awareness: 4 Most Dangerous Food Allergies and How You Can Avoid a Reaction," Medical Daily, May 13, 2014, http://www .medicaldaily.com/food-allergy-awareness-4-most-dangerous-food -allergies-and-how-you-can-avoid-reaction-282206.

26   richer countries, on average: George Du Toit, Yitzhak Katz, Peter Sasieni, David Mesher, Soheila J. Maleki, Helen R. Fisher, Adam T. Fox, et al., "Early Consumption of Peanuts in Infancy Is Associated with a Low Prevalence of Peanut Allergy," Jounal of Allergy and Clinical Immunology 122, no. 5 (2008): 984–91, http://dx.doi.org/10.1016/j.jaci.2008.08.039.

26   developing countries seem to be catching up: Prescott et al., "A Global Survey."

27   decrease in vitamin D levels across many populations: Peter J. Vuillermin, Anne-Louise Ponsonby, Andrew S. Kemp, and Katrina Allen, "Potential Links Between the Emerging Risk Factors for Food Allergy and Vitamin D Status." Clinical and Experimental Allergy 43, no. 6 (2013): 599–607.

27   Allergy rates increase: Allen and Koplin, "Theories," 123–33.

27   This latitude trend: Steve Simpson Jr., Leigh Blizzard, Petr Otahal, Ingrid Van der Mei, and Bruce Taylor, "Latitude Is Significantly Associated with the Prevalence of Multiple Sclerosis: A Meta-Analysis," Journal of Neurology, Neurosurgery, and Psychiatry 82, no. 10 (October 2011): 1132–41, doi:10.1136/jnnp.2011.240432; Robert Amato, Michele Pinelli, Antonella Monticelli, Gennaro Miele, and Sergio Cocozza, "Schizophrenia and Vitamin D Related Genes Could Have Been Subject to Latitude-Driven Adaptation," BMC Evolutionary Biology 10 (2010): 351, http://www.biomedcentral.com/1471–2148/10/351; and Paul Knekt, Annamari Kilkkinen, Harri Rissanen, Jukka Marniemi, Katri Sääksjärvi, and Markku Heliövaara, "Serum Vitamin D and the Risk of Parkinson's Disease," Archives of Neurology 67, no. 7 (2010): 808–11, http://doi.org/10.1001/archneurol.2010.120.

27   more likely to have an autumn or winter birthday: Milo F. Vassallo, Aleena Banerji, Susan A. Rudders, Sunday Clark, Raymond

J. Mullins, and Carlos A. Camargo Jr., "Season of Birth Is Associated with Food Allergy in Children," *Annals of Allergy, Asthma and Immunology* 104, no. 4 (2010): 307–13, doi:10.1016/j.anai.2010.01.019.

27   in the northernmost states: Carlos A. Camargo Jr., Sunday Clark, Michael S. Kaplan, Philip Lieberman, and Robert A. Wood, "Regional Differences in EpiPen Prescriptions in the United States," *Journal of Allergy and Clinical Immunology* 120, no. 1 (2006): 131–36.

28   in populations with high incidence of skin cancer: Ibid.

28   a study undertaken in Australia: Nicholas J. Osborne, Obioha C. Ukoumunne, Melissa Wake, and Katrina J. Allen, "Prevalence of Eczema and Food Allergy Is Associated with Latitude in Australia." *Journal of Allergy and Clinical Immunology* 129, no. 3 (2012): 865–67.

28   blood samples were taken: Katrina J. Allen, Jennifer J. Koplin, Anne-Louise Ponsonby, Lyle C. Gurrin, Melissa Wake, Peter Vuillermin, Pamela Martin, et al., "Vitamin D Insufficiency Is Associated with Challenge-Proven Food Allergy in Infants," *Journal of Allergy and Clinical Immunology* 13, no. 4 (2013): 1109–16.

28   Mechanistic data: Allen and Koplin, "Theories," 123–33; and Margherita T. Cantorna and Brett D. Mahon, "Mounting Evidence for Vitamin D as an Environmental Factor Affecting Autoimmune Disease Prevalence," *Experimental Biology and Medicine* 29, no. 11 (2004): 1136–42.

29   vitamin D supplementation: Matthias Wjst, "Another Explanation for the Low Allergy Rate in the Rural Alpine Foothills," *Clinical and Molecular Allergy* 3 (2005): 7; Joshua D. Milner, Daniel M. Stein, Robert McCarter, and Rachel Y. Moon, "Early Infant Multivitamin Supplementation Is Associated with Increased Risk for Food Allergy and Asthma," *Pediatrics* 114 (2004): 27–32, http://pediatrics.aap publications.org/content/114/1/27; and Elina Hyppönen, Ulla Sovio, Matthias Wjst, Swatee Patel, Juha Pekkanen, Anne-Liisa Hartikainen, and Margo Riitta Järvelinb, "Infant Vitamin D Supplementation and Allergic Conditions in Adulthood—Northern Finland Birth Cohort 1966," *Annals of the New York Academy of Sciences* 1037 (2004): 84–95, doi:10.1196/annals.1337.013.

29   The so-called hygiene hypothesis: Rob Dunn, "Eating off the Floor: How Clean Living Is Bad for You," *Scientific American* guest blog, January 29, 2012, http://blogs.scientificamerican.com/guest

-blog/eating-off-the-floor-how-clean-living-is-bad-for-you; and Jerome Groopman, "The Peanut Puzzle: Could the Conventional Wisdom on Children and Allergies Be Wrong?" *New Yorker*, Feb. 7, 2011, http://www.newyorker.com/magazine/2011/02/07/the-peanut-puzzle.

30   If kittens do not receive: John Douglas Pettigrew, "The Effect of Visual Experience on the Development of Stimulus Specificity by Kitten Cortical Neurones," *Journal of Physiology* 237 (1974): 49–74.

30   critical period for the infant immune system: Sally F. Bloomfield, Ros Stanwell-Smith, and Graham A. Rook, "The Hygiene Hypothesis and Its Implications for Home Hygiene, Lifestyle and Public Health: Summary," report by the International Scientific Forum on Home Hygiene, 2012, http://www.ifh-homehygiene.org/best-practice-review/hygiene-hypothesis-and-its-implications-home-hygiene-lifestyle-and-public.

30   old friends: Mei Wang, Caroline Karlsson, Crister Olsson, Ingegerd Adlerberth, Agnes E. Wold, David P. Strachan, Paolo M. Martricardi, et al., "Reduced Diversity in the Early Faecal Microbiota of Infants with Atopic Eczema," *Journal of Allergy and Clinical Immunology* 121 (2008):129–34; and Hans Bisgaard, Nan Li, Klaus Bonnelykke, Bo Lund Krogsgaard Chawes, Thomas Skov, Georg Paludan-Müller, Jakob Stokholm, et al., "Reduced Diversity of the Intestinal Microbiota During Infancy Is Associated with Increased Risk of Allergic Disease at School Age," *Journal of Allergy and Clinical Immunology* 128, no. 3 (2011): 646–72, doi:10.1016/j.jaci.2011.04.060.

31   having older siblings: Wilfried Karmaus and Calin Botezan, "Does a Higher Number of Siblings Protect Against the Development of Allergy and Asthma? A Review," *Journal of Epidemiology and Community Health* 56, no. 3 (March 2002): 209–17.

31   owning a pet dog (but not a cat): Claudio Pelucchi, Carlotta Galeone, Jean-François Bach, Carlo La Vecchia, and Liliane Chatenoud, "Pet Exposure and Risk of Atopic Dermatitis at the Pediatric Age: A Meta-Analysis of Birth Cohort Studies," *Journal of Allergy and Clinical Immunology* 132, no. 3 (2013): 616–22, http://dx.doi.org/10.1016/j.jaci.2013.04.009.

31   other studies of kids growing up: Melanie Thernstrom, "The Allergy Buster: Can a Radical New Treatment Save Children with

Severe Food Allergies?" *New York Times*, March 7, 2013, http://nyti
.ms/VGhjpP.

31   Farm kids do seem: Duncan Graham-Rowe, "Lifestyle:
When Allergies Go West," *Nature* 479 (November 24, 2011): S2
–S4, doi:10.1038/479S2a; and Sabina Illi, Martin Depner, Jon Genu-
neit, Elisabeth Horak, Georg Loss, Christine Strunz-Lehner, Gisela
Büchele, et al., "Protection from Childhood Asthma and Allergy in
Alpine Farm Environments—the GABRIEL Advanced Studies," *Jour-
nal of Allergy and Clinical Immunology* 129, no. 6 (2012): 1470–77.

31   top theories for the rise: Hikaru Okada, Chantal Kuhn, Hélène
Feillet, and Jean-François Bach, "The 'Hygiene Hypothesis' for Autoimmune and Allergic Diseases: An Update," *Clinical and Experimental Immunology* 160 (2010): 1–9; and Stefan Ehlars and Stefan
H. E. Kaufman, "Infection, Inflammation, and Chronic Diseases:
Consequences of a Modern Lifestyle," *Trends in Immunology* 31, no. 5
(2010): 184–90, doi:10.1016/j.it.2010.02.003.

32   eating significant quantities of hydrogenated oils: Merryn
J. Netting, Philippa F. Middleton, and Maria Makrides, "Does Maternal Diet During Pregnancy and Lactation Affect Outcomes in Off-
spring? A Systematic Review of Food-Based Approaches," *Nutrition*
30, no. 11 (2014): 1225–41.

32   diets high in fresh produce: Leda Chatzi and Manolis Kogevi-
nas, "Prenatal and Childhood Mediterranean Diet and the Development of Asthma and Allergies in Children," *Public Health Nutrition*
12, no. 9A (2009): 1629–34, doi:10.1017/S1368980009990474; and
Netting et al., "Does Maternal Diet," 1225–41.

32   Cigarettes or possibly other environmental toxins: Junenette
L. Peters, Renée Boynton-Jarrett, and Megan Sandel, "Prenatal Environmental Factors Influencing IgE Levels, Atopy and Early Asthma,"
Current Opinion in Allergy and Clinical Immunology, 13, no. 2 (2013):
187–92, doi:10.1097/ACI.0b013e32835e82d3; and Philippe Bégin
and Kari C. Nadeau, "Epigenetic Regulation of Asthma and Allergic Disease," *Allergy, Asthma and Clinical Immunology* 10 (2014): 27,
doi:10.1186/1710-1492-10-27.

33   "contaminated by confounding": Allen and Koplin, "Theories,"
123–33.

33   Delaying the introduction of eggs: Jennifer J. Koplin, Nicholas J. Osborne, Melissa Wake, Pamela E. Martin, Lyle C. Gurrin, Marnie N. Robinson, Dean Tey, et al., "Can Early Introduction of Egg Prevent Egg Allergy in Infants? A Population-Based Study," *Journal of Allergy and Clinical Immunology* 126, no. 4 (2010): 807–13.

33   Delaying the introduction of cereal grain: Jill A. Poole, Kathy Barriga, Donald Y. Leung, Michelle Hoffman, George S. Eisenbarth, Marian Rewers, and Jill M. Norris, "Timing of Initial Exposure to Cereal Grains and the Risk of Wheat Allergy," *Pediatrics* 117 (2006): 2175–82.

33   regular fish consumption: Inger Kull, Anna Bergstrom, Gunilla Lilja, Goran Pershagen, and Magnus Wickman, "Fish Consumption During the First Year of Life and Development of Allergic Diseases During Childhood," *Allergy* 61 (2006): 1009–15.

35   In mice, placing egg white or peanut proteins: Joachim Saloga, Harald Renz, Gary L. Larsen, and Erwin W. Gelfand, "Increased Airways Responsiveness in Mice Depends on Local Challenge with Antigen," *American Journal of Respiratory and Critical Care Medicine* 149 (1994): 65–70, doi:10.1164/ajrccm.149.1.8111600; and Jessica Strid, Jonathan Hourihane, Ian Kimber, Robin Callard, and Stephan Strobel, "Disruption of the Stratum Corneum Allows Potent Epicutaneous Immunization with Protein Antigens Resulting in a Dominant Systemic Th2 Response," *European Journal of Immunology* 34 (2004): 2100–9, doi:10.1002/eji.200425196.

35   In humans, food allergen–specific T cells: Frank C. van Reijsen, Abraham Felius, Erik A. K. Wauters, Carla A. F. M. Bruijnzeel-Koomen, and Stef J. Koppelman, "T-Cell Reactivity for a Peanut-Derived Epitope in the Skin of a Young Infant with Atopic Dermatitis," *Journal of Allergy and Clinical Immunology* 101 (1998): 207–9. http://dx.doi.org/10.1016/S0091-6749(98)70410-5.

35   inflamed skin was treated: Gideon Lack, Deborah Fox, Kate Northstone, and Jean Golding for the Avon Longitudinal Study of Parents and Children Study Team, "Factors Associated with the Development of Peanut Allergy in Childhood," *New England Journal of Medicine* 348 (2003): 977–85, doi:10.1056/NEJMoa013536.

36   explains a lot of the geographical differences: Gideon Lack, "Update on Risk Factors for Food Allergy," *Journal of Allergy and Clinical Immunology* 129 (2012): 1187–97.

36   In countries in Africa and Asia: Robin Green and Davis Luyt, "Clinical Characteristics of Childhood Asthmatics in Johannesburg," *South African Medical Journal* 87, no. 7 (1997): 878–82; David J. Hill, Clifford S. Hosking, Chen Yu Zhie, Roland Leung, Karmen Baratwidjaja, Yoji Iikura, Nagalingam Iyngkaran, et al., "The Frequency of Food Allergy in Australia and Asia," *Environmental Toxicology and Pharmacology* 4, nos. 1–2 (1997): 101–10; Gideon Lack, "Epidemiologic Risks for Food Allergy," *Journal of Allergy and Clinical Immunology* 121 (2008): 1331–36; and Bee Wah Lee, Lynette Pei-Chei Shek, Irvin Francis A. Gerez, Shu E. Soh, and Hugo P. Van Bever, "Food Allergy—Lessons from Asia," *World Allergy Organization Journal* 1 (2008): 129–33, doi:10.1097/WOX .0b013e31817b7431.

36   Geography can also affect the severity: Andrea Vereda, Marianne van Hage, Staffan Ahlstedt, Maria Dolores Ibañez, Javier Cuesta-Herranz, Jenny van Odijk, Magnus Wickman, et al., "Peanut Allergy: Clinical and Immunologic Differences Among Patients from 3 Different Geographic Regions," *Journal of Allergy and Clinical Immunology* 127, no. 3 (2011): 603–7, doi:10.1016/j .jaci.2010.09.010.

36   Including the study of ten thousand: Du Toit et al., "Early Consumption," 984–91, http://dx.doi.org/10.1016/j.jaci.2008.08.039.

37   having well-educated parents: Lene Hammer-Helmich, Allen Linneberg, Simon Francis Thomsen, and Charlotte Glümer, "Association Between Parental Socioeconomic Position and Prevalence of Asthma, Atopic Eczema and Hay Fever in Children," *Scandinavian Journal of Public Health* 42, no. 2 (2014): 120–7, doi:10.1177/1403494813505727; Andrea S. Weber and Gerald Haidinger, "The Prevalence of Atopic Dermatitis in Children Is Influenced by Their Parents' Education: Results of Two Cross-Sectional Studies Conducted in Upper Austria," *Pediatric Allergy and Immunology* 21, no. 7 (2010): 1028–3, doi:10.1111/j.1399–3038.2010.01030.x; and Sarah A. Taylor-Black, Harshna Mehta, Elisabete Weiderpass, Paolo Boffetta, Scott H. Sicherer, and Julie Wang. "Prevalence of Food Allergy in New York City School Children," *Annals of Allergy, Asthma and Immunology* 112, no. 6 (2014): 554–56, doi:10.1016/j .anai.2014.03.020.

38   Zoe had to call the paramedics: Zoe Duncan, mother of Raphael, Lockland, and Meredith, in discussion with author, May 19, 2015.

Chapter 2: The Solution

41   "something like three hands shot up": Jerome Groopman, "The Peanut Puzzle: Could the Conventional Wisdom on Children and Allergies Be Wrong?" *New Yorker*, February 7, 2011, http://www.newyorker.com/magazine/2011/02/07/the-peanut-puzzle.

41   observational study of ten thousand Jewish children: George Du Toit, Yitzhak Katz, Peter Sasieni, David Mesher, Soheila J. Maleki, Helen R. Fisher, Adam T. Fox, et al., "Early Consumption of Peanuts in Infancy Is Associated with a Low Prevalence of Peanut Allergy," *Journal of Allergy and Clinical Immunology* 122, no. 5 (2008): 984–91, http://dx.doi.org/10.1016/j.jaci.2008.08.039.

42   countries in Asia and Africa: Robin Green and Davis Luyt, "Clinical Characteristics of Childhood Asthmatics in Johannesburg," *South African Medical Journal* 87, no. 7 (1997): 878–82; David J. Hill, Clifford S. Hosking, Chen Yu Zhie, Roland Leung, Karmen Baratwidjaja, Yoji Iikura, N. Iyngkaran, et al., "The Frequency of Food Allergy in Australia and Asia," *Environmental Toxicology and Pharmacology* 4, nos. 1–2 (1997): 101–10; Gideon Lack, "Epidemiologic Risks for Food Allergy," *Journal of Allergy and Clinical Immunology* 121 (2008): 1331–36; and Bee Wah Lee, Lynette Pei-Chei Shek, Irvin Francis A. Gerez, Shu E. Soh, and Hugo P. Van Bever, "Food Allergy—Lessons from Asia," *World Allergy Organization Journal* 1 (2008): 129–33, doi:10.1097/WOX.0b013e31817b7431.

42   American Academy of Allergy, Asthma and Immunology: David M. Fleischer, Jonathan M. Spergel, Amal H. Assa'ad, and Jacqueline A. Pongracic, "Primary Prevention of Allergic Disease Through Nutritional Interventions: Guidelines for Healthcare Professionals," *Journal of Allergy and Clinical Immunology: In Practice* 1 (2013): 29–36, http://www.jaci-inpractice.org/article/S2213-2198(12)00014-1/fulltext.

43   Learning Early about Peanut: George Du Toit, Graham Roberts, Peter H. Sayre, Henry T. Bahnson, Suzana Radulovic, Alexandra F. Santos, Helen A. Brough, et al., "Randomized Trial of Peanut Consumption in Infants at Risk for Peanut Allergy," *New England Journal of Medicine* 372, no. 9 (2015): 803–13.

43   A follow-up study, LEAP-On: George Du Toit, Peter H. Sayre, Graham Roberts, Michelle L. Sever, Kaitie Lawson, Henry T. Bahnson, Helen A. Brough, et al., "Effect of Avoidance on Peanut Allergy after Early Peanut Consumption," *New England Journal of Medicine* 374 (2016): 1435–43, doi:10.1056/NEJMoa1514209.

43   interim advice was offered: Rebecca Gruchalla and Hugh A. Sampson, "Preventing Peanut Allergy Through Early Consumption—Ready for Prime Time?" *New England Journal of Medicine* 372, no. 9 (2015): 875–77.

43   as early as three months of age: Gideon Lack, head of the Children's Allergy Service at Guy's and St. Thomas's NHS Foundation Trust and professor of pediatric allergy at King's College London, in discussion with the author, April 28, 2015.

43   The second of such studies: Michael R. Perkin, Kirsty Logan, Anna Tseng, Bunmi Raji, Salma Ayis, Janet Peacock, Helen Brough, et al., "Randomized Trial of Introduction of Allergenic Foods in Breast-Fed Infants," *New England Journal of Medicine* 374 (2016): 1733–43, doi:10.1056/NEJMoa1514210.

45   most parents have been needlessly avoiding: James Baker, CEO and chief medical officer of Food Allergy Research and Education, in discussion with the author, March 29, 2016.

48   "People should understand that it is not their fault": Ibid.

48   consensus on "interim guidelines": David M. Fleischer, Scott Sicherer, Matthew Greenhawt, Dianne Campbell, Edmond Chan, Antonella Muraro, Susanne Halken, et al., "Consensus Communication on Early Peanut Introduction and the Prevention of Peanut Allergy in High-Risk Infants," *Pediatrics* 136, no. 3 (2015): 600–604. http://www.jacionline.org/article/   S0091–6749%2815%2900785-X /full.

48   the broader recommendations: David M. Fleischer, Jonathan M. Spergel, Amal H. Assa'ad, and Jacqueline A. Pongracic, "Primary Prevention of Allergic Disease Through Nutritional Interventions: Guidelines for Healthcare Professionals," *Journal of Allergy and Clinical Immunology: In Practice* 1 (2013): 29–36, http://www.jaci -inpractice.org/article/S2213–2198(12)00014-1/fulltext.

49   attaching peanut proteins: Charles B. Smarr, Chia-Lin Hsu, Adam J. Byrne, Stephen D. Miller, and Paul J. Bryce, "Antigen-Fixed

Leukocytes Tolerize Th2 Responses in Mouse Models of Allergy," *Journal of Immunology* 187 (2011): 5090–98, doi:10.4049/jimmunol .1100608.

49   Nadeau had medical-grade flours: Whitney Morgan Block, lead study coordinator for FARE Center of Excellence, Stanford University, Stanford, CA, email messages, including study materials, sent to author, April 28 and May 5, 2016.

52   "Food allergies amplify": Melanie Thernstrom, "The Allergy Buster: Can a Radical New Treatment Save Children with Severe Food Allergies?" *New York Times*, March 7, 2013, http://nyti.ms /VGhjpP.

52   through an epigenetic twist: Philippe Bégin and Kari C. Nadeau, "Epigenetic Regulation of Asthma and Allergic Disease," Allergy, Asthma & Clinical Immunology 10 (2014): 27, doi:10.1186/1710 -1492-10-27.

Chapter 3: Implementing at Home

56   wiped with birth canal bacteria: Maria G. Dominguez-Bello, Kassandra M. De Jesus-Laboy, Nan Shen, Laura M. Cox, Amnon Amir, Antonio Gonzalez, Nicholas A Bokulich, et al., "Partial Restoration of the Microbiota of Cesarean-Born Infants via Vaginal Microbial Transfer," *Nature Medicine* 22 (2016): 250–53, doi:10.1038 /nm.4039.

57   The research on breast-feeding: Melanie C. Matheson, Katrina J. Allen, and Mimi L. K. Tang, "Understanding the Evidence For and Against the Role of Breastfeeding in Allergy Prevention," *Clinical and Experimental Allergy* 42 (2012): 827–51; and Debra de Silva, Matthew Geromi, Susanne Halken, Arne Host, Sukhmeet S. Panesar, Antonella Muraro, Thomas Werfel, et al., "Primary Prevention of Food Allergy in Children and Adults: Systematic Review," *Allergy* 69 (2014): 581–89, doi:10.1111/all.12334.

57   breast-feeding has been associated: Jane Allen and Debra Hector, "Benefits of Breastfeeding," *New South Wales Public Health Bulletin* 16, no. 4 (2005): 42–46; Cesar G. Victora, Bernardo Lessa Horta, Christian Loret de Mola, Luciana Quevedo, Ricardo Tavares Pinheiro, Denise P. Gigante, Helen Gonçalves, et al., "Association Between Breastfeeding and Intelligence, Educational Attainment, and Income at 30 Years of Age: A Prospective Birth Cohort Study

from Brazil," *Lancet* 3, no. 4 (2015): e199–e205, doi:http://dx.doi .org/10.1016/S2214–109X(15)70002–1; and Robin Nixon, "Breast Milk Does DNA Good," *LiveScience*, May 22, 2010, http://www.live science.com/6498-breast-milk-dna-good.html.

63   4 percent of babies: Fiona McAndrew, Jane Thompson, Lydia Fellows, Alice Large, Mark Speed, and Mary J. Renfrew, "Infant Feeding Survey 2010" (Leeds, England: Health and Social Care Information Centre, 2012).

63   no adverse effects on breast-feeding duration: Michael R. Perkin, Kirsty Logan, Tom Marrs, Suzana Radulovic, Joanna Craven, Carsten Flohr, and Gideon Lack on behalf of the EAT Study Team. "Enquiring About Tolerance (EAT) study: Feasibility of an Early Allergenic Food Introduction Regimen," *Journal of Allergy and Clinical Immunology* 137, no. 5 (2016): 1477–86, http://dx.doi.org/10.1016/j .jaci.2015.12.1322.

69   "When the joy goes out of eating": Ellyn Satter, *Secrets of Feeding a Healthy Family: How to Eat, How to Raise Good Eaters, How to Cook* (Madison, WI: Kelcy Press, 2008).

70   researchers have found: Leann L. Birch, Susan L. Johnson, Graciela Andresen, John C. Peters, and Marcia C. Schulte, "The Variability of Young Children's Energy Intake," *New England Journal of Medicine* 324, no. 4 (1991): 232–35; and Clara M. Davis, "Results of the Self-Selection of Diets by Young Children," *Canadian Medical Association Journal* 41, no. 3 (1939): 257–61.

71   Even the pickiest eaters: Robin Nixon, "Grown Up but Eat Like a Kid?" *LiveScience*, syndicated to NBC. November 28, 2010, http:// www.nbcnews.com/id/40357712/ns/health-diet_and_nutrition/# .VykHtWNqec8.

73   if kids regularly ate peanuts: George Du Toit, Peter H. Sayre, Graham Roberts, Michelle L. Sever, Kaitie Lawson, Henry T. Bahnson, Helen A. Brough, et al., "Effect of Avoidance on Peanut Allergy after Early Peanut Consumption," *New England Journal of Medicine* 374 (2016): 1435–43, doi:10.1056/NEJMoa1514209.

Chapter 4: Prevention
81   the best strategy: George Du Toit, Graham Roberts, Peter H. Sayre, Henry T. Bahnson, Suzana Radulovic, Alexandra F. Santos,

Helen A. Brough, et al., "Randomized Trial of Peanut Consumption in Infants at Risk for Peanut Allergy," *New England Journal of Medicine* 372, no. 9 (2015): 803–13; George Du Toit, Peter H. Sayre, Graham Roberts, Michelle L. Sever, Kaitie Lawson, Henry T. Bahnson, Helen A. Brough, et al., "Effect of Avoidance on Peanut Allergy After Early Peanut Consumption," *New England Journal of Medicine* 374 (2016): 1435–43, doi:10.1056/NEJMoa1514209; David M. Fleischer, Scott Sicherer, Matthew Greenhawt, Dianne Campbell, Edmond Chan, Antonella Muraro, Susanne Halken, et al., "Consensus Communication on Early Peanut Introduction and the Prevention of Peanut Allergy in High-Risk Infants," *Pediatrics* 136, no. 3 (2015): 600–604, http://www.jacionline.org/article/ S0091-6749%2815%2900785-X /full; David M. Fleischer, Jonathan M. Spergel, Amal H. Assa'ad, and Jacqueline A. Pongracic, "Primary Prevention of Allergic Disease Through Nutritional Interventions: Guidelines for Healthcare Professionals," *Journal of Allergy and Clinical Immunology: In Practice* 1 (2013): 29–36, http://www.jaci-inpractice.org/article/S2213 -2198(12)00014-1/fulltext; and Michael R. Perkin, Kirsty Logan, Anna Tseng, Bunmi Raji, Salma Ayis, Janet Peacock, Helen Brough, et al., "Randomized Trial of Introduction of Allergenic Foods in Breast-Fed Infants," *New England Journal of Medicine* 374 (2016): 1733–43, doi:10.1056/NEJMoa1514210.

General Index

age categories, 10–11
    pregnancy through newborn,
        56–58
    three to five months, 58–60
    five to nine months, 65–66
    nine to twelve months, 67–69
    one to three years old, 69 72
    three to five years old, 72–74
Allen, Katrina J., 33
allergen avoidance. *See* avoiding
    allergens
allergen exposure. *See* early
    exposure to allergens
allergist, consultation with, 12,
    50 51, 55
*Allergy, Asthma and Clinical
    Immunology*, 32
allergy tests, 12, 59–60. *See also*
    skin-prick tests
almond butter, 133
    recipe, 133–34
    weekly guidelines, 62, 87
almond flour, 87–88, 135
    recipe, 135–36
almonds, 31–32, 74, 76–77, 88
American Academy of Allergy,
    Asthma and Immunology
    (AAAAI), 26, 42–43, 48
American Academy of Pediatrics
    (AAP), 42, 48
amount of food, 81–82. *See also*
    weekly guidelines
Amsterdam, Elana, 137

anaphylaxis, 18, 21, 49
animals, 31
"arsenic eaters of Styria," 20–21
asthma, 25–26
Austria, "arsenic eaters of Styria,"
    20–21
autoimmune disorders, increase
    in, 4–5
autumn birthday, and food
    allergies, 27–28
avoiding allergens, 2, 3–4, 31–33,
    41–43
    Henry's case, 1–4

baby fat, 58
baby's attention, catching, 61
baby's cues, responding to, 58
baby setting the pace, 62–63
baby's swallowing technique, 60
bacterial colonization, 56–57
Baker, James, 25–26, 45, 48
Bamba, 42
banana allergy prevention, 95–96
bisphenol A (BPA), 61, 91
blood tests
    author's case, 4
    Clara's case, 18, 19
Brazil nuts, 38, 76, 89
bread, 71, 78, 82, 93, 94. *See also*
    wheat allergy prevention; *and*
    Recipe Index
    weekly guidelines, 62, 82, 94,
        182

Recipe Index